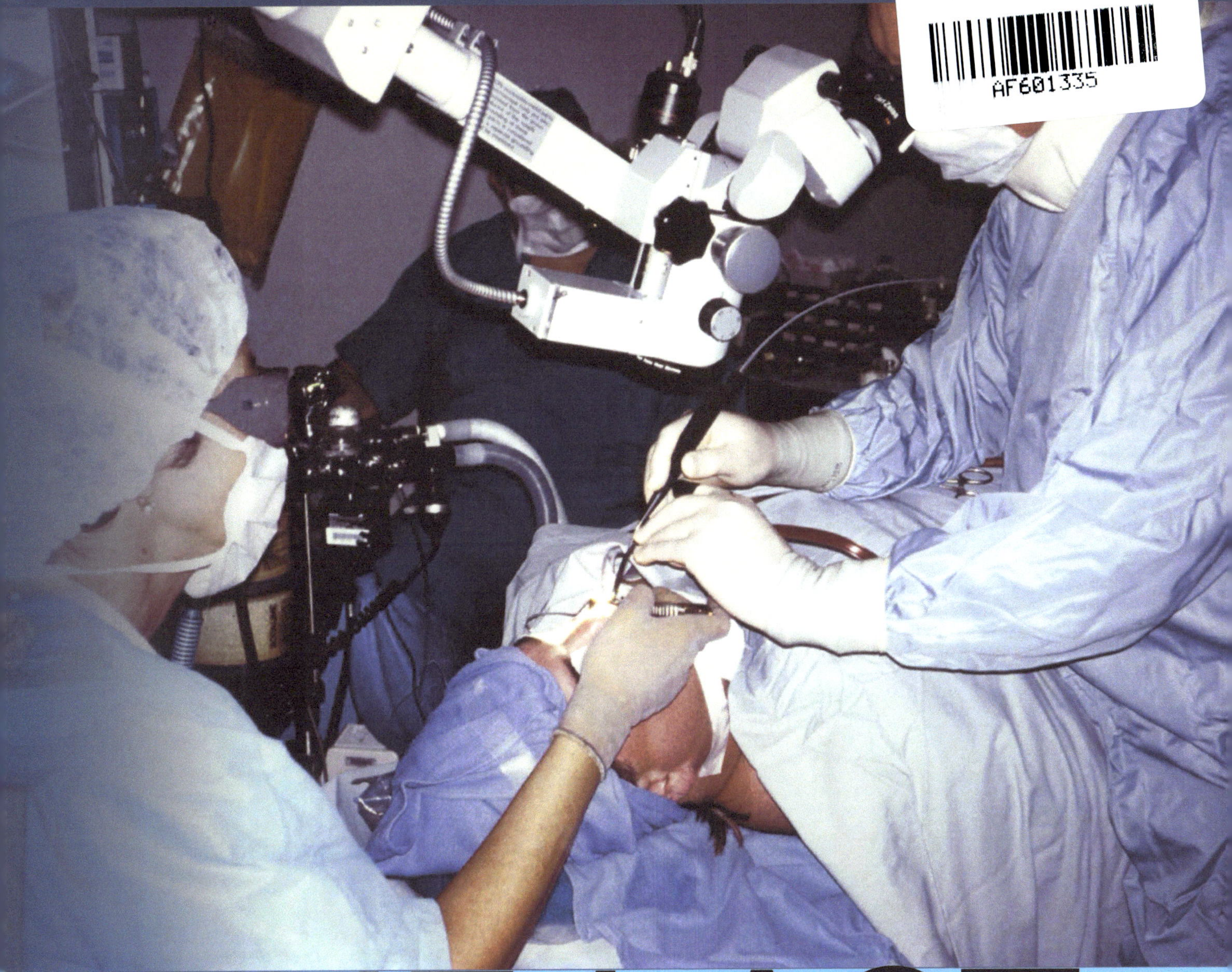

THE LAST SURGEON

LEWIS NEWBERG, MD

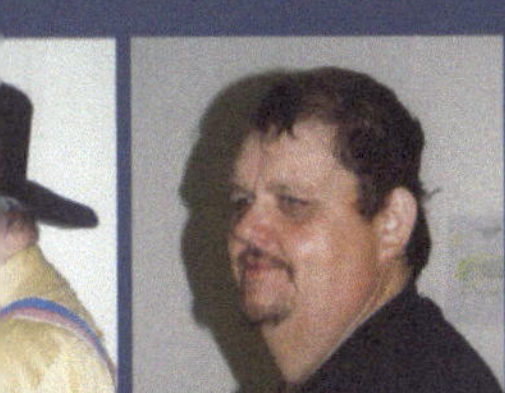
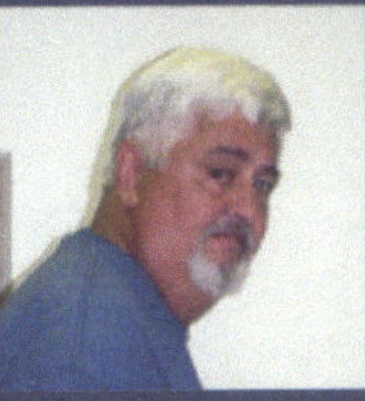
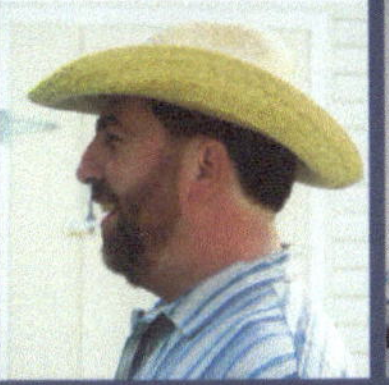
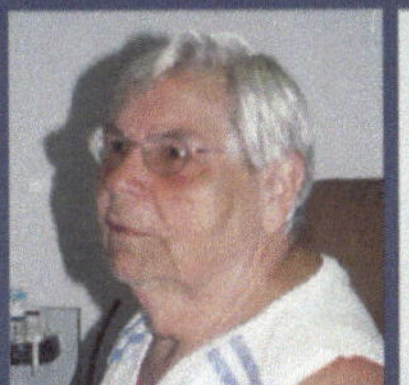
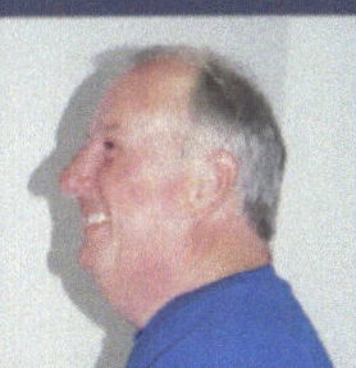
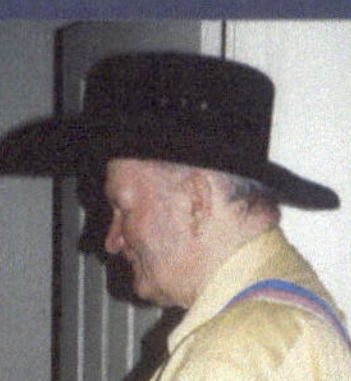
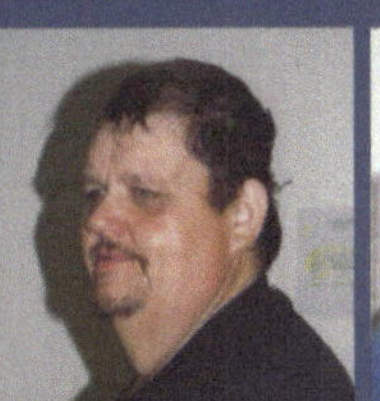

Library of Congress Control Number: 2008907519
ISBN: Softcover 978-1-4363-6508-6
Hardcover 978-1-4363-6509-3

This book was printed in the United States of America.

To order additional copies of this book, contact:
Xlibris Corporation
1-888-795-4274
www.Xlibris.com
Orders@Xlibris.com

TABLE OF CONTENTS

ACKNOWLEDGEMENTS

Nurses of Philipsburg Hospital

Michelle Amerman	RN	Michelle
Christa Maney	RN	"Crista Galli"
Jolene Dudak	RN	Jolene
Susanne Cram	RN	Sue

Secretaries

Kim Yable – interviewing pt's for study; keeping my head plugged on
Cathy Hanson
Lynn Shimmel

Administrators of Philipsburg Hospital

Mikhael Kennedy	Mike Loomis	Karen Blair

Physicians

Larry Adams MD – GP/Internist

Anesthesiologist

Andrew Glickman MD Andy; the best I'ved worked with over 40 plus years; died 2008 of complications in sleep apnea.

Special people-special thanks for their support

Representative Bud George
John Wozniak—State Senator
Board of Trustees — each and every one

Friends and Heros

Stan Lewis M.D. died Nam 1961 Air-CAV
Stanley Everett MD Pediatrician
Toby Everett

PROLOGUE:

MY NEVER-ENDING ADVENTURE STORY

We were an improbable pair. I was young, he was old. He loved science and I pursued English. Out of touch with the times, he made archaic allusions that I only sometimes got—and when he referenced anything in pop culture, his brow furrowed in confusion. But, despite this, sitting at that coffee table, we had one thing in common—he had a story to tell. And I was going to write it.

When Dr. Lewis Newberg first asked me to translate his book to the world, I was skeptical of myself. I was barely a junior in college, glancing over this man's life work. I felt suddenly and acutely just how young I was. Looking down at the material he handed me over coffee, I was further confused what exactly my job was—the meticulously hand written pages were in English.

"I write like a scientist," he told me. "You have to turn into a human."

Working through his writings, I soon understood. He handed me a lab report and I had to turn it into a story. He gave me facts that I had to interweave in a tale. Some how, despite of our differences, I had to take his words and tell them my way.

But somewhere, skimming through his loose—leaf draft, I uncovered his secret. In between the numbers and underneath the biology, there was the greater actuality. A man who spent his life, risked his license, and dedicated a career to fighing for the few. A man who discovered an anwer to the impossible—found a cure for the incurable. Fiction couldn't write itself this beautiful. Legends would never be repeated as good.

I never heard of sleep apnea—knew nothing of its side affects, the causes, the treatments. My first introduction to sleep apnea took place on a rainy Friday morning over coffee, meeting with the man who had struggled with it throughout his hife.

Calm and frank, brown eyes tiredly met mine.

"I have sleep apnea," he told me. "And I will die from it."

Over coffee, through e-mails, and even a letter now and then, Dr. Lewis Newberg sent me his life. And I present it to you, an improbable pair—his story and my words.

CHAPTER 1

The Kosher Chicken

Evolution of dactyls and birds produced chickens
Plump kosher chickens for a Jewish kitchen
Chicken plumage causes an allergic rash
Uncle Charlie plucked the feathers in a flash
Feather pillows aren't orthopedic
There's a wholesale switch to tempurpedic

The Permian – Triassic extinctive event 250 million years ago was an ice age blip in geologic time. The end of the Permian period showed that the roach was the king of the insects; at this time pterosaur's made its way into the skies. This flying reptile was leathery and a meat eater. Domestication of the pterosaurs, called a Dactyl, introduced a gamey source of meat with a "wild" chicken taste. An enterprising franchise operator of restaurants in Jurassic Park cross-bred the Dactyl with a bird. This sparrow paired well with the Dactyl. They fell in love. The offspring were large chickens and the chicken-dino combo first appeared in the Jurassic Park menu. The hadrosaur hamburger with trimming completed a menu well suited for Raptors and T-rex. The burgers were cooked rare; real rare. Blood filled the bottom of the plates as natural gravy.

There was no clue, no warning, when a meteorite hit the Yucatan 65 million years ago. This KT extinction was in the late cretaceous period. The lights in Jurassic park went out; permanently. The cozy intimate relationship of the taxonomic groupings of bird and reptile decreased. The absence of fossil evidence was the Lazarus taxon and followed one of the "Big Five" extinctive events of all time. The new and related species, the "Kosher Chicken" appeared in fossils. This resurrection of missing species can be identified from snippets and fragments of RNA and DNA. The evolution of a species disappearing from fossil records, only to reappear is the Lazarus taxon. The dactyl and birds from evolution of the chicken disappeared.

The "Phoenix", the mystical bird that never dies, represents a capacity for vision and a new beginning. We know that the Phoenix, at the end of its life cycle, burns itself in a nest of cinnamon twigs. The new young phoenix has a rebirth of life. The big bird flies ahead, scanning the future. The species known as kosher chicken, suddenly reappeared in nature. This phenomenon of resurrection was first discovered in South East Asia. Fossilized bones of Kung-pao chicken were found in a pot in China. Szechuan chicken was to spread far and wide to all the continents on Planet Earth. There's a lesson to be learned in the expansion of homo sapiens (man). It may be nothing more than accidental continental drift from movements of the tectonic plates.

I spent summers in Fleichmanns, New York, a small town in the Catskill Mountains. The family killed kosher chickens. Uncle Charlie was a devoted and designated chicken maven. He was in charge of dispatching chickens. Normally, Rabbi's, kosher butchers or those with a kosher union label are the legal authorities to kosher chickens. My job at the farm was Chairman of the "Bagging and Disposal of Feather" committee. I was a teenage feather picker! The feathers were collected in burlap bags for removal. Charlie knew the dietary laws, and the humane way to kill and bleed chickens. A painless, quick knife cut into the throat followed by removal of feathers and evisceration of the organs and guts were quick. Cold, clean brook water from a surrounding Catskill stream finished the cleaning process. The smell test was confirmatory for "sweet-meat." The fresh, fleshy yellow color ensured a perfect pot. Grandma would always say "my chickens are clean."

Grandma Essie, who emigrated from Europe to the United States in the early twentieth century, didn't give a hoot for the convergent evolution theory. Her need was the kosher chicken fitting into the pot. No feet, neck, wings, beaks or eyeballs would hang over the lid. The golden yellow broth in the pot was medicinal. Many people knew the golden brew contained natural liquid penicillin. Most people were ignorant that the broth supplied essential ingredients to the immune system. My father swore soup was a hemorrhoid shrinker and lubricant. She would skin the schmaltz (fat) from the surface of her chilled refrigerator soup. She didn't know from coronary artery disease. Grandma was always right. There's nothing else to know. Kosher chicken served on the Sabbath is not only salvation; its tradition. Like it says in the eleventh commandment, "For my family that loves us, God made the kosher chicken."

I became an unemployed feather picker after the family moved form Fleichmanns into Queens, New York. No longer do feathers cause my major problems with allergies and asthma. Synthetic fibers in bedding followed by Tempurpedic synthetic materials changed everything. After KT extinction wiped out animal life, repopulation of Planet Earth took place before Columbus and Magellan sailed the seas. The winds and tides were treacherous in the Pacific, chickens boarding transport ships, including the Kon Tiki, for the Americas and Europe was dangerous. The Polynesian oceanic islands were refueling stops in the migration. Corn kernels, bugs, earthworms and water were packed into barrels. There was rumor of hanky-panky with red waterfowl in American Samoa; this was hushed up. This "mass migration" of flightless sea birds produced a big flying bird. The late Cretaceous area fossils show gene segments of an albatross. The albatross was a good luck omen flying over the fleet. Its diet of squid vomit from whales didn't steal food from the boat chickens. But a cook's mate shot down the albatross and bad luck haunted the H.M.S. Kosher Chicken. Shish kabob recipes decimated the chicken population. Many chickens jumped ship as penance for killing the albatross.

Evolutionary biology of the immune system would develop in the "Bursa of Fabricus" of young chickens. B cells (B lymphocytes) that produce antibodies have been located in their shoulder sacs. The immunity of Jewish chicken soup has a scientific derivation.

The meteorite that rendered the kosher chicken and dinosaurs extinct was a major ecologic disaster. The age of mammals and the biologic evolution of a newer, smaller and fatter kosher chicken began. A cottage tourist industry sprang up in the 12 mile Chicxulub crater. This 12 mile wide crater is recognized as the ideal Mexican vacation spot for couples who like to stare into a hole. The locals refer to the spot of the meteorite as "the tail of the devil." There are road signs advertising "home of the dino-burger." The recent Yucatan Hilton shows posters that the Kentucky Fried Chicken (KFC) logo was of Cretaceous, and not Madison Avenue origin. There are two statues at the entrance of the town eulogizing the founding fathers. There is the Archaeopteryx (dactyl) holding hands with a kosher chicken. The franchises surrounding the crater have good taste. A great, great relative from the Jurassic Park operation runs the show.

CHAPTER 2

Planet Schmutz

Particles, particles everywhere cause the sneeze
Floating schmutz in the breeze
Winds that were invisible
Become clearly visible
Pollens and pollutants up the nose
Boogers shaped like a garden hose
Large molecules cause the sneeze
Subatomic antigens trigger the wheeze
Snoring and gasping with out a clue
Waiting and watching the morning dew
Mirror mirror on the wall
Who cures them all?

Always one to encourage a vivid imagination, Mom told me planet clean existed long ago in a far away galaxy. Particles of dirt floated upwards to mimic Saturn's rings, Planet Schmutz turned Planet Earth's daylight into night. At age thirteen, Mom appealed to my love for comic books. I was a freckled adolescent with glasses convinced I would save the world. Pollution became an intergalactic battle for me. I turned smog into Lex Luther, and clean air legislation to Batman. It wasn't the fireflies in the night air, it was dangerous particles every where. She described the atmospheric blight as a tsunami of biblical proportions descending on our home. In my mind, I convinced myself that I alone could stop them.

My curiosity in childhood was discussed with mom and dad. Dad drove the family to Grandma Essie's house and small farm in the Catskills. While dad navigated the dusty highway of old Route 28, I poked my head through the space between the seats. Pushing a pair of slightly crooked glasses up my nose, I barely paused between questions. Demanding the answers to my many queries, my behaviour crossed the obnoxious boundary.

Terminally carsick on the trip to Fleischmann's, the "nerd" label was borne at roadside pit stops. It was my first battlefield commission. It took five or six roadside stops to navigate the one hundred and forty mile trip. The family stop for the use of a restroom at a gas station gave me extra time to sneak and explore the area. There were luscious blackberries growing in the back for a gourmet treat. Fooled them. Ate the berries. Ten minutes later, another car stop for a gross emptying maneuver. The nerd label was changed to the logo "loser." Dad was hot! Mother was not! Her first borne son and future doctor could do no wrong. Barfing at the side of the road was distinctly unpleasant. This was a teaching call for self-discipline.

As a young child, the Catskills had almost a pure, untainted quality to me. Awakening earlier than the rest of the house, I'd creep outside to bring in glass bottles of milk delivered on the porch. I always lingered longer than necessary while gathering up the bottles. The air was crystal clear and the morning dew had clean water vapor. The surrounding atmospheric winds were invisible. You could wear a white shirt without ring around the collar. I learned that a two toned black collar and white shirt is not a fashion statement. It's a filthy shirt. Remembering the pristine purity of Fleischmann's air, I asked Mom, "where has all the clean air gone."

We lived in the big house near the railroad tracks. Fleischmann's was a small town in upstate New York named from the "Margarine" family. Grandma Essie cooked on a large wood burning stove. A stove pipe was more than adequate to remove smoke and ash. The air was clean. We could always open a window. The top grate was removed by a curved iron bar. It worked well if a tad slow. It was heavy!

A coal furnace in the basement heated our house. A coal bin carried fuel by conveyor belt through an open window. A half-moon shaped funnel separated the pieces of coal by size. Gravity worked quite well to fill the pails; a coal shovel did the rest. In the morning, dad removed the ashes.

Dad's move into New York City for employment became permanent. Oil furnaces heated room radiators. Electricity or natural gas was used to cook. New York Cities airborne particulate matter from coal, oil and gasoline was increasing. Industrialization from coal-fire power plants, metal and chemical industries and the natural pollutants were building up.

It seemed that large particles (antigens, allergens) and subatomic fragments present different breathing problems. I'll try to stop the science talk. I'm supposed to be a doctor who doesn't talk like one. The small fragments, like cigarette smoke bypass the nose and enter the lung. If antigenic, or if an irritant, an immune response is elicited. A wheeze or cough is triggered, asthma or bronchitis is born. My mother's two pack-a-day cigarette habit over forty years caused both wheezing and cough. Eventually, and inevitably, shortness of breath caused her death from emphysema. The bandits that snuffed out her life were the coal tars, microscopic dust, and particulate matter in ciggies. Like any good superhero, I was out for the best for mom and my patients. Just try telling mom to stop smoking. But a super hero's mom is the one woman who ranks above him. She said, "cram it."

Sleep apnea was never a concern for her. She was superthin. She could never understand the fuss over exercise and diet. Fribbles, oversized fries and greasy hamburgers were staples in my diet over fifty years. And can you blame me. They tasted really good. OSA was never a concern to me; until I got it.

Small atmospheric particles, floating in the breeze provoke a response in the sinus tissues. The immune responses to processing these foreign antigens are like a dysfunctional pinball machine. These responses cause autoimmune diseases. For example, sleep apnea and the metabolic syndrome which include coronary artery disease. The autoimmune-like kissing cousins you know lived on your block. Maybe he has an obnoxious dog, maybe he never takes out the trash—but once you discover him, you wish to God you hadn't.

But the irony was that, in the end, pollution wasn't my Mom's main enemy. Everyday for thirty years, Mom didn't help her health by smoking two packs of cigarettes. Wondering about the big fuss over lack of exercise and eating French fries, she died of emphysema. Sleep apnea was never a concern for her or me.

Along with the freckles and glasses, I developed allergies as a youngster and started allergy shots from age ten. They helped symptoms of rhinitis (my own nickname for a runny nose), itchy eyes, and the allergic salute. The sleeve of my T-shirt was a definite bail out maneuver. A loud throaty sneeze was the hallmark symptom of allergy—spring and fall—I would scare away every little girl in my class with one loud, resounding "Ach-ho!" Every year, various medications: antihistamines, steroid nasal sprays and air conditioning made life tolerable—both for me and the easily frightened girls.

With this experienced background in allergies, I was chosen for Ear, Nose, and Throat residency in Milwaukee. Marquette University had a four-year program that prepared me for a general practice. Entering private practice in Baltimore after serving the Coast Guard during the Vietnam conflict, life looked as simple as it once did to me, picking up the milk bottle in the Catskills. But, as cliché as it sounds—things don't always turn out as you think. Being curious, suspicious, and somewhat irreverent, my practice was limited to obstructive sleep apnea (OSA).

Age ten and my allergies were bad. The "allergic salute" was my universal sign. It wasn't meant for public display. The loud throaty sneeze couldn't be hidden. A cardinal sign and symptom of spring and fall allergies. I would scare away every little girl in my class with one loud resounding "sneeze-honk."

Little relief of symptoms from allergy medication prompted my parents to seek an allergy specialist. Fifty years ago, my doctor skin-tested using tooth picks to scratch the skin as a prelude to placing a small amount of antigenic extract. Redness and spider-leg extensions of a positive reaction were easy to see and measure. My mixture of allergy extracts, mainly mites, dust, some fungi and most pollens, was used in a solution for desenitization. This has been my on/off method for 60 years. Little did I know, at the age of ten, that the antigen in the shot would stimulate a blocking antibody against the allergy antibody anchored to a mast cell. One antibody blocked another. Activation and release of histamines could not take place. My testing showed significant skin reactions; actually quite impressive. The wheal and flare reaction on my upper arm was severe to cause swelling of all the pollen test sites. This impressive response is the 4 t reaction; dosage with antigens start at very dilute concentrations. Sterilizers were used to prevent contamination of needles from repeated use. Disposable needles hadn't arrived yet. The pollens that dive-bombed into my nose to penetrate the ethmoid mucus layer and lay waste to the surface sinus cells would now face a reved up adaptive immune system protected by blocking antibody. The treatment worked well enough. The sneeze-honk disappeared. Wallah, all the girls were attracted back.

CHAPTER 3

Mom's Dream

Immune cells in embryonic muck
Differentiation into stem cells wasn't luck
Liver and spleen cells moving into bone marrow
The whole caboodle moved in a wheel barrel
Her first son in the oven
She was absolutely driven
With the birth of Doctor Wonderful
The bris was quite colorful

My nature to question everything about this, and that, started early in embryonic life. My intrauterine fidgeting led to a lifelong "nudgering" habit. But mother seized the day. Her dream was educating doctor boychuk from the get go. She had a plan to alter fetal I. Q. development. Supposedly, funneling classical music into her belly button would create sound wave vibrations traveling south via my umbilical cord. Her messages of communication were to bypass the skin and amniotic fluid barriers. Mozart and Beethoven via telepathy was the beginning of many cockeyed schemes. Another gesture was singing "La Cucaracha", the "roach song" in her shower. This was the crude attempt to teach Spanish. Then there was imprinting telepathic signals into my brain using the method and techniques of bright strobe lights. She used a 75 watt light bulb to the music of "YMCA". This was her adaptation to imprinting the brain waves exhibited in "Close Encounters of the Third Kind". Alas, my brain failed to pick up this worthless gaggle. Spanish remained alien. However, my medical specialization into Ear Nose and Throat was supplemented with allergy sub-specialization. I noticed the roach antigen in my box of inhalant allergy extracts. Perhaps a message did get through.

My I. Q. never increased. A lack of communication between mother and I would last a lifetime. My response was to get even. An opportunistic kick started the conflict. A drop kick, followed by a free kick was getting to her. The rugby kick caused retaliation. Her message was "shut up, quiet down and suck on your yolk sac . . . or else." Being good wasn't easy. What pressure. An intrauterine fetal panic attack in the first trimester can be serious. An emergency 911 call to report this felony. It would be hard to diagnose a pattern. There were no witnesses to confirm my charges. However the assault at the bris had many observers. There was a definite threat.

The outline of my immune system required lymph nodes for processing messages of the cells. A cytokine nanonetwork (CNN) to cover signals to and from the immune system was introduced. The pluripotent all-seeing stem cell was in place and supported by fillers of soft mushy bone marrow tissues. The cells filled the marrow like a jelly donut. This stromal or mesenchymal filler would churn out white cells to do their thing. Many years later, the fat tissue and marrow would differentiate into fat cells and produce the hormone Leptin. The marrow was like a beehive. Surface proteins that would differentiate types of cells, organ maturity and all kinds of precursors would be the "Cluster of Differentiation" (CD) numbering system.

My nine month vacation with mother reminded me of evolution. Loss of my great ancestor's tail and closure of my gill slits allowed me to breathe better. The thought of being the only child in class able to swing from a tree, or live in a goldfish bowl is a nightmare.

Admonished by mom that if the violence and kicking directed to her didn't quiet down, I would become a chicken. Already cursed with freckles and glasses, a beak and feather would damage my image further. A horrific thought was the idea of crackpot chicken fricassee. My life preserver, the umbilical cord, saved me from the thought of the coming separation anxiety.

My yolk sac was the earliest sign of sleep-disordered breathing. You try sleeping from the top of a uterus upside down! My yolk sac hung down to my knees . . . . Hanging from the top of mom's uterus like an aromatic duck, I was naked and defenseless. My belly protruded like a hanging chad. Thank you, mother for not changing me into a chicken. My embryonic life was brief; but stressful.

Primitive stem cells infiltrated the liver and spleen. They started functioning at two months. Even their form as donut shaped cells wasn't classy for Mom. She wasn't pleased with the neighborhood and engineered the move to an uptown address with a better zip code. This permanent move to the bone marrow took place at 7 months. And not a second too long! This term of endearment to every parent is chiseled into rock . . ."are we there yet, are we there yet?"

Now 23 pairs of chromosomes, 35,000 genes and 3 billion base pairs of amino acids would have every immune response covered. An integrated immune system for all eventualities in the future would result in the innate and adaptive defense systems. Organs, tissues, cells, molecules and atomic matter would continue to organize and shape future immune inflammatory responses.

The birth of doctor "wonderful" was uneventful. My first uttered word was "gimme", but it could've been "momma." Thank God it wasn't "cluck-cluck." There was a whole lot of shaking (me) at the bris. Yelling and crying at the circumcision confirmed loss of a body part. This adventure is the beginning of the greatest story ever told.

CHAPTER 4

Seeds of Sleep Apnea

Natural allergens in the air
Contaminated by pollutants up there
Dickens wrote about big, fat Joe
He moved so-so slow
Snoring started the craze
First step in the sleep apnea phase

Sucking on my yolk sac real hard prevented my development into a kosher chicken. Luckily mom was right. It was still a horrific thought.

My childhood flirtation with sleep apnea can be examined in historical text. I was a precocious nerd, and tales of London always fascinated me. The Tower, Elizabeth, Henry VIII and Harrods are unique. My Jack Russell terrier is named Henry.

The industrial revolution is credited to England. Trees were plentiful, and wood was the cheap commodity. Centuries of cutting down trees with increased prices was cramping industrial growth. The next cheap plentiful source of energy was sea coal. Large deposits from the Carboniferous period powered heating homes and energy needs for factories. A sea change in the atmospheric pollution mix was soot particles and hydrocarbons joining naturally occurring particles like pollens.

In the early 1900's, the Four Horsemen of the Apocalypse reappeared. This fearsome, gruesome foursome was wood, coal, oil and gasoline. London was to witness a dimming of sunlight. A haze was to cover the city. Gradual darkening of the day worsened with temperature inversions. Smoke and London fog became "SMOG." The word stuck. Eventually a "Big Smoke" affected London in 1952. This "Great London Smog" killed 12 thousand Londoners.

Parliament started to get the message. Hotsy-totsy Lords and M.P.'s were getting sick. The atmospheric "cocktail" effects of ozone, and volatile oil compounds (VOC) made shopping at Harrods uncomfortable. Victims of sulfur dioxide (SO_2) and nitrous oxide (NO_2) were plotzing over. The morgues became overcrowded. London was fast becoming a laboratory covered by a dark, particulate cloud. Rats had better survival rates than shoppers. Flying into Heathrow was an occupational hazard.

The politicians passed the Clean Air act. To show their pain and empathy to the public they raised the price of petrol for their Rolls Royce's. Of course, all anti-pollution legislation for industry was grandfathered in. No pain, no gain. And the fat lady sang "Casey would waltz with the Strawberry blonde, and the band played on." And the death rates increased exponentially.

Immunity began with the birth of Paul Ehrlich in 1854. He was born into a Jewish family in Poland. His province became part of Germany. Not surprising from a Jewish background, (take myself for example), Paul pursued medicine. He won the Nobel Prize in 1908 for his work in immunology. He opened new doors to the unknown. He worked with the microscope in cellular pathology. His work in immunology overlapped with his other interests. Paul discovered "das Mastzellen," commonly known among friends as the mast cell. I came to dislike this "purple people eating cell" resembling a hemorrhoid. It causes sleep apnea.

I, on the other hand, was Lewis Newberg MD, "American Nebisher!". The first born son into a Jewish family in the Bronx, NYC in 1939. Mother was a full time homemaker. Dad busted his chops at full throttle every week. He was the "candy man." Being a candy broker after going bust as a manufacturer took a full effort to put food on the table. A son, who like Paul Ehrlich was destined for greatness. Well, the twenty-first century form of greatness. The only thing I was destined to win was a divorce settlement. Thinking about it now . . . what a loser.

Not quite akin to Ehrlich, I was destined to spend quality time studying mast cells. My nerd instincts and intellect was particularly well suited to this exciting subject. My luck peaked with uncovering the existence of mast cells in three OSA patients. Ethmoid sinus tissue in OSA was key to a new hypothesis in sleep apnea. The flooding of ethmoid (sinus) tissue with mast cells was a unique and sentinel finding. It's found in no other ethmoid disease states. Even ethmoid infections and polyps don't exhibit mast cells as the only acute cell. Mast cells are known for the immune response of pollens. Let me appease your curiosity right now. How you wonder? Sleep apnea is a disease of molecular medicine.

Sleep apnea presented a wake-up call to Charles Dickens. The inspiration for the Dickens character of Joe, "Big Fat Joe" in the "Posthumus Papers for the Pickwick Club." Joe fell asleep knocking at the door. He stood there, the eighth wonder of the world. Joe was snoring and unconscious while standing. Arousable with a little poking, severe mental dullness was obvious. Dickens was the catalyst to show the effects of the environment causing sleep apnea.

Years later "Fat Joe" appeared in scientific literature. The medical world was introduced to the "Pickwickian Syndrome"; Joe was the poster boy. The article proposed a spinach salad as treatment. Diet and exercise emanated hope to all sufferers of OSA. Unfortunately, this disease doesn't respond to spinach salads, or exercise, or gastric bypass surgery. This disease grew to be the 600 pound gorilla on the block.

Jefferson Hahn, patient number six of the magnificent seven (see photos) was a Pickwickian. Jeff's disease had progressed to the stage of respiratory and cardiac failure, which required daily oxygen. Spinach salad didn't do the trick either.

CHAPTER 5

Ancestry of Sleep Apnea

Bacteria and fungi filled the seas
Fossils and amber were the keys
Plate tectonics and Continental drift
Caused the North American rift
Weirdo arthropodic segmented Trilobites
Crawled onto the land to evolve Dust mites

The Big Bang 13.7 billion years ago (bya) was more than a College party. This event, the creation of the universe, was real important because the large rotating cloud of rocks and gas gave birth to our solar system 4.5 billion years ago. Two simple gases, hydrogen and helium would send neutrons, protons and electrons to orbit the nucleus. We stole other elements from surrounding stars. Carbon was so important. We are carbon based life forms. Nuclear fusion of hydrogen into helium would ignite the star into our sun. The structure of all molecules is determined by the size of matter.

It is the special distortion of matter that allows photons to diffuse out in an atom. The interconnections between subatomic particles lead to the strong ionic and chemical gradients in the molecule. Gravity, magnetic forces, dust particles, other elements and radiation including cosmic rays separated Earth and the planets into a series of rings around the sun.

Early Earth was molten. The earth's surface hardened into a solid crust. Earth expanded with an atmosphere of methane, ammonia and other green house gases. Small amounts of oxygen were bound to hydrogen or other minerals on the surface. There was no place on the surface for my mother to "light up." She wouldn't survive nicotine deprivation. Photosynthesis was coming online; oxygen increased. The coming ozone layer and the beginnings of unicellular life did support combustion.

4 billion years ago a molecule appeared from a chance collision of atoms with overlapping electrons. This electron cloud would establish probability patterns. The subatomic interrelationships gained the ability to replicate itself. The modern replicator, DNA, evolved from a simple unicellular cell to the multi cellular level. Gene fragments developed the many sizes and shaped living organisms. With the beginning of simple life, some real doozies developed. This highly elaborate scheme has lasted through the rock and roll era. Extinctive events throughout geologic history have not stopped the advance in civilization. The evolution of an immune defense system is efficient in preserving our life. Unfortunately the cellular and protein immune responses to foreign substances, has proven detrimental to OSA. Plate tectonics and continental drift would split North America from Asia and Europe. The Atlantic and Pacific oceans would usher in the Devonian period 400 million years ago. The Devonian explosion of life fed off temperate climates and lots of oxygen. Snowball Earth, followed by the Devonian explosion of plant and animal life became an extinctive happening with the Great Dying. This Permian—Triassic (PTr) occurred 250 million years ago. From 800-250 million years ago two distinct ice age periods decimated many marine, plant and terrestrial vertebrate species.

Weird, sucking "opalina" arthropodic fish look-like vacuum cleaners. These mobile Oreck's remove debris from the sea floor. They see from "4 eyes" that protrude. The word "4 eyes" evolved to mainstream language usage in the twentieth century. Trilobites, a 3-segmented arthropodic fish with three lobes appeared first in the Cambrian period (800 million years ago) but had disappeared early in the Devonian period. They were disappearing before the PTr extinctive phase as new predators developed to eat trilobites. They disappeared but not before introducing a working trilobite onto land. The land locked arthropods were resurrected as the dust mite.

Steam escaped into the atmosphere from the crusts volcanic activity. The formations of clouds rained to form the oceans. The volcano's produced high energy emissions to drive chemical reactions to produce more complex cells. The first cell 3.5 billion years ago was generic. A covering cell membrane contained a phospholipid bi-layer bubble. Proteins and carbohydrates in the cell would serve various functions in regulating the passage of material through the membrane and in reacting to the environment. There was absence of a nucleus but DNA was its genetic code. RNA was used for information transfer and protein synthesis. Enzymes were the energy catalyst for reactions. All living cells would have DNA except viruses and prions.

Extinctive geological events like ice ages and meteorites did not stop progress in development of the immune system. And Earth didn't miss a beat in the development to survive to better days! The immune system took billions of years to advance.

3 billion years ago photosynthesis evolved. Plentiful CO_2 and H_2O were the raw materials. The energy of sunlight from UV and cosmic radiation produced energy rich carbohydrates.

It was the stimulation of some oxygen by incoming radiation that created the ozone layer. O2 became O3 (ozone) with the addition of the oxygen atom. The oxygen produced as a waste product. Actually, the first one-celled life form was an explorer looking for a better life. Any life was better than breathing a poisonous gas. Unicellular organism is good. This overachiever was to become multi-cellular and take on various tasks. At the time, 2 billion years ago, bacteria joined and a DNA virus gave birth to the nucleus. Life was good. The oceans became warm and algae plants and fungi grew at the waters edge. These life forms, the cyanobacteria made oxygen. Oxygen would displace methane. Methane is a potent greenhouse gas which kept Planet Earth warm. Temperatures plummeted and "snowball earth" ushered in the first ice age. The only survivors of life were deep sea marine unicellular life forms.

Volcanic activity was to form a single land mass of Rhodinia. But the buildup of greenhouse gases under the ice continued. Volcanic activity exploded with release of poisonous gases. The single land mass of Rhodinia split apart into the super continent of Pangea 250 million years ago.

Sun ripened algae and bacteria took refuge among volcanic rocks. The cyanobacteria turned the oceans green—photosynthesis was the "in" thing. Well-preserved fossils are found in the Burgess Shale fauna. They have been located in the Canadian Rockies. The Burgess Shales in Yunnan Province, China contains fossils similar to the Burgess.

The cyanobacteria are living fossils. These bacteria growing in volcanic rocks are stromatolites, Earths oldest fossils. They form limestone and are known as "sea biscuits." Modern stromatolites were first discovered in Shark Bay, Australia in 1956. The stromatolites are nothing special to write home about, but some of the tourist attractions are quite lively. Driving the outback highway to Western Australia, one can pick up genuine limestone stromatolites to outline a sports field. Take home a few bags or buy the live stromatolite plants in Gia National Park. Gia plants are popular.

The local sport fishing store rents diving equipment. Shark Bay is famous for the view of the Whale Shark. This endangered species enters the bay in July to breed, and eat plankton.

On the other hand Carchavodon Carcharius, the Great White grows to 20 feet with 5,000 pounds of love. It loves cheeseburgers decorated with surf boards and flippers. It shows up anytime. The Great Whites prefer prey with high energy content of fat. Schools fatten up at Shark Island in preparation for the migration to the waters off Miami Beach. Renting a spear gun and encountering a White will bring an adrenalin rush. A shark cage is just no fun. Fish for them in the wild and give them a chance. The sports store have all kinds of torn flippers and fragmented surf boards for sale. The Missing Persons Bureau at Shark Island is very busy. The sharks get bigger and fatter each day. This Howdy-Doody show is a daily event. Many tourists miss their flights home. I wonder why?

The Devonian period was witness to a bewildering humongous fungus. Called prototaxites, it was classified as a tree. It turns out that prototaxites was stem-like. No leaves, no roots, no flowers; just stems. It was the largest knows Devonian organism. 400 million years later, this living fossil was discovered alive and well, producing button mushrooms in Crystal Falls, Michigan.

The Crystal Falls Business Association saw the opportunity for the tourist trade. The "Humongous Fungus Festival" became a yearly event. The Fungus Fudge, Fungus Burgers and Fungus Tee Shirts were copycats of the Jurassic Park amusement park. The Fungus Burger is covered with authentic prototaxites button mushrooms. It's said to taste like a kosher chicken with a sanitized clean smell.

It has taken 10,000 years to poison the atmosphere. We have failed as caretakers of Planet Earth. Natural and artificially created pollution produced airborne emissions. Methane gas and ammonia once covered the earth to protect us from UV radiation. Loss of the ozone layer would expose the planet to cosmic rays. The changes in the greenhouse gases resemble prehistoric gaseous atmospheric levels. In spite of passing laws, the continual bombardment will require drastic action. The populace could move underground, or fly away to another planet or air-condition the Earth. Those antigens in my allergy extract testing kit include bacteria, fungi, cockroach and dust mites. Their body parts including organs and waste are in solution. They may survive, perhaps in spore form. He who laughs last, laughs best.

CHAPTER 6

Galen

Galen divided medicine into four humours
Imbalances in the vapors wasn't a rumor
Blaming the throat for OSA is just wrong
It's mast cells and hormones playing a snore song
OSA is organs, tissues, cells and molecules
His four humours are open to ridicule

Shamanism was a doctor between the natural and spiritual world. The sleep spirits and interpretation of dreams by the shaman required special knowledge. Full time rituals and spiritual associations were precursors to physicians, medical societies and institutions. The earliest sleep-disordered breathing patterns—evil spirits—were treated by voodoo doctors.

Voodoo medicine and the science of medicine were to clash. The evil spirits causing sleep apnea was developing traction. It took a great medical leader to abolish the ideas of witch doctors. Hippocrates characterized ragweed allergy, and OSA as a health issue. Writings from 400 BC were to eulogize Hippocrates as the Father of Medicine, and King of the Sneeze. Hippocrates was the first scientist that taught every disease had only natural causes. It was Galen who plagiarized Hippocratic writings in the abundance of the four humours in the body.

Galen ripped off the hypothesis of earth, fire, water and air. The basic imbalance was poisonous vapors in the air. This idea of excesses of the hot air, from particles in the air, was the cause of OSA. This air, as one of the four essential humours, was identified as future Captain Planet powers as well!

According to Galen (and here's where he was off his rocker), the thrust of treatment was reducing harmful surpluses of humours. Blood and hot air imbalances. Bah! Humbug!

Excessive sweet odors were detected in Galen's abundant "hot air" vapor. He traced these fragrances to flowers. He coined the word pheromone or sex hormone; to the flowering pimpernel. He looked here, he looked there, but it was the damned elusive scarlet pimpernel. Eating or smelling these "roses" didn't provide the answer to reduce the humors. Frustrated, he singled out the "Big Red" flower and plant, the Rambutan. The red fruit was difficult to locate as a "Where's Waldo" cartoon. Galen's fruity odor vapor theory was as big a success story as the vapors. Galen came up with zip (nada, niente, nothing) in the treatment of OSA.

It was back to the drawing board for this giant in medicine. It would take multiple leeches to treat the excessive vapors in obese OSA patients. He was a pioneer in building leech farms. Cross breeding led to humongous leeches that could treat many OSA cases with one application. The octopus tentacle leech was a genetic breakthrough. It was the eighth wonder of the world watching a leech with multiple suction cups suck on six OSA patients. Galen was to decrease the cost of medicine. He also advertised with Humphrey Bogart in the movie "African Queen." He showed off his prime "big black" beauties that could suck 40%

more blood. Humphrey Bogart was the purveyor of these show-leeches and would receive residuals for many years.

There was a pandemic in OSA cases and Galen rose to the challenge. Instead of leeches, he domesticated giant bats and vampires in Transylvania. These suckers could really get the Kool-aid flowing quickly. He also found out that leeches could be placed onto the swollen tonsils to reduce their size. His discovery of the scarlet pimpernel, and Rambutan would lead to the observation of beautiful, plump, red, granulated mast cells in ethmoid tissue. He was the first scientist to see the connection between flowers and pollens and sleep apnea. His leech reductions were the prelude to the modern throat surgery espoused by Doctor Ikematsu in the 20th century.

Scientists introduced the medical word "dipstick" to his character. His non-sensical rantings turned off the medical society. His last studies saluted ancestral worship and the divination of fortune telling patterns in tea leaves. He was big on séances, Ouija boards and communication from ghosts and spirits. He left specific instructions for Voodoo incantations directed to were removed by repeated episodes of blood letting. Leeches were in short supply. They were as scarce and difficult to locate as a werewolf with sharp canines. Galen looked world-wide, and analyzed this, and studied that. A leech farm and industry sprang up in Transylvania. Blood letting, emetics and venipuncture created the sucking sound of a thirsty leech. OSA patients were subject to primitive methods of treatment. Obsolete technology of dirty scalpels and used needles were added to off-the-wall algorithms to diagnose and treat OSA.

Kosher chickens used in blood rituals were regulated. They must have feathers, breathe and take a minimum sound of one "cluck". He was a procurer of voodoo Barbie dolls for Wal-mart. The insurance companies wouldn't pay for the leech treatments. The medical procedure falls into a category of cosmetic surgery.

There is a scientific and intellectual demand for observable facts to sustain a scientific theory. The hypothesis that OSA is a dysfunction of the vapors has not stood the test of time. The medical societies willingness to perpetuate shibboleths is part of institutional craziness. The wacky professors hypothesize OSA is an anatomical disease of throat tissue obstructions and negative upper airway pressures. No matter what? This nonsense goes on. The captain Marvel comic book poked fun in the Marvel universe.

The four vapors of Galen lived on as perpetrators of scientific knowledge. There was a new concept of a flowing river Styx in the nose between atmospheric air and the ethmoid cellular layer. This river is a liquid stream of mucus. The ancients described the river of death. The (mucus) carrying dead and dying ragweed. Golden rod pollen had a ripe, very sweet pungent odor. A ferryman (Charon) carried antigens (souls) from Earth (nasal air), to and from Hades (sinus cells). These dead antigens can really build up crusts. Finger action or blowing ones nose, would clear the pond.

Actually, Galen was a loser; too much of the weed! He didn't have a clue. The vapor imbalance, became the Four Horsemen of the Apocalypse; War, pestilence, famine and death. I suppose that Galens vapors theory did point to the Four Horsemen of the Apocalypse. Galen wasn't far off in determining four causes. Updating my four causes of OSA just a bit, to something more like Big Mac's, oversized fries, Coca-Cola, and lack of exercise. These four no-no's didn't mean much during my residency in the 1960's. Today's "Four Horsemen of the Apocalypse" are immortalized in film. The backfield of the fighting Irish is a metaphor corresponding to the four elements of immunity: organs, tissues, cells and molecules including subatomic particles.

Modern thought of the origin of OSA centered about the anatomy of the throat—a part of the body most people don't give much thought to. (Which is understandable—how many times have you heard someone say, "She's beautiful. She has a great . . . . anatomy of the throat"?) Tonsils, some big, some small, and/or uvula/soft palates that are dysfunctional. They are frequently worn out like flabby socks. At night, the throat tissues fall backwards to block the upper airway. The tissues flail in the wind. The normal air currents from nose to throat into trachea are increased nightly. Hammering the throat tissues changes the pressure differentials. Negative pressures become stronger and this unnatural phenomenon continues.

Oxygen levels fall and OSA intervenes. The excessive daytime sleepiness starts the tailgate party. The parking lot activates a block party and eventually the bedroom scene. Blankets are thrown off, breathing stops for variable periods of time and the "gasp" to open up the airway. All this happens while asleep. Wives suffer waiting for the next breath.

The elite medical establishment expanded the physician base to include internists and sleep study experts. There is a sleep lab in every block and University Centre. Since the surgical treatment of OSA was a total flop, the medical treatment expanded exponentially. The CPAP (constant positive airway pressure), machine became the gold standard in medical treatment. Elite Rockefeller, Howard Hughes and John Hopkins institutes failed me. OSA confuses the experts. Billions are spent for research and the "boys" can't get their act together. They failed me. It seems that Galen came as close thousands of years ago. Clearly, OSA is not chopped liver . . . it's very serious.

The backbone of modern medicine is institutionalized. Residency training and filling out grants for research projects in OSA should lead to success. The modern in's and out's of getting grants is kinda like Flesh Gordon enjoying the pleasures in the many caves of Mongo. And if you're not one of the academics elite pets; no funding. Suck-up 101 and brown-nosing 102 are two mandatory college requirements for research. How silly of me to think that excellence in medicine is represented by Golden Institution Committee. Actually, I don't remember many prizes to a committee for medical excellence. Always felt the Nobel Prize to an individual physician-scientist benefited mankind the most.

At Jabberwocky University, the sleep study specialist hooks up patients to CPAP machines. They are very important doctors; they carry beepers. Thus doctor Beeper teaches survivalist medicine with an old iron-lung technique revised downward to a small bedside unit. This upper airway splint (CPAP) uses positive pressure to breathe for the patient. The sleep apnea machine raises blood oxygen and relieves daytime sleepiness. The other signs and symptoms in OSA aren't touched; patients will continue with their high blood pressure pills and digitalis.

Doctor Beeper, met doctor Quack. The surgical approach to remove flabby throat tissue and cure snoring and sleep apnea has been unsuccessful. Ahah! If removing big floppy hangy tonsils and the soft palate/uvula doesn't work, what about strengthening the tissues? In the land of Jabberwocky, things are strange indeed. An so two famous scientists, Drs. Beeper and Quack developed the "BQ" holodeck program for all space cadets. In the puzzle palace of the University Medical Centre, things are not what they seem.

The injection of tissue glue, or at the insurances industries biding, the less expensive Krazy Glue. Liquid cement into the tonsil dries quickly overnight. The hardness and drying period of the glue is markedly reduced using the hair dryer. Building a scaffold from an erector set seems a positive way to go.

Perhaps throat tissues need more bulk and strength; Small steel struts in the configuration of rungs of a ladder. Known as the "Hook and Ladder" operation, it was well received by the American Academy. Did the University boys finally cure snoring/sleep apnea. Wrong! The operation was quietly downgraded in the scientific literature to showing "promise." The only positive finding was the rapid extrusion of the plastic and steel. They could be spit out quite nicely. The only flaw in the operation was failure. The throat post-operatively looks like a destroyed munitions dump of scrap metal. The surgeries failed me. The surgeries failed the public. Bye-the-way; where did all the billions go?

The mast cell crawls in. The mast cell crawls out of ethmoid tissue. The humoral immunity in the adaptive immune system is the switching of antibodies that anchor to the mast cell. There is immune response of B and T lymphocytes to nasal inflammation. The production of proteins to coat B and T cells, and an adaptability to respond by humoral and cell-mediated anti bodies, cytokines and hormones. This allows great diversity in function. The production of complex neuropeptides (hormones) from blueprints are the stuff immune diseases are associated with. The rise and fall of OSA will depend on examining the genetics and environmental markers in the immune system. We've come a long way since Galen. Or have we? The 4th horseman is the pale rider; death! It's congestive heart and/or respiratory failure. Its this or that, one way or the other. The beginning of modern medicine, from Hippocrates to Galen was only seven or eight hundred years. Two thousands years later, medicine slowly recovered. From Satanism through the patent medicine craze in the 1800's; it's been slow going.

Nature hides its secrets well. The clues to a disease are usually obscured until exposed. In OSA, the vector doesn't seem to be a bacteria, virus or insect. Scientists are in a way like detectives. Perhaps they are not as glamorous as Sherlock Holmes but their basic science investigations are essential in identifying the culprit. Graduate students and research money fund these innovations. In OSA, the unearthing of red, glamorous mast cells in ethmoid tissue was dumb luck. These red cells light up like shiny sequins. The fictional super villains included the "Four Riders of the Dark." The "bandit" that rob's everyone with OSA can blame the culprit – the super-villainous mast cell. Please read on.

CHAPTER 7

The Young Surgeon

The operating room nurses know quality work
They won't pick a dork
They recognize young surgeon adaptation
Better than acting with constipation
The young surgeon operates without emotion
Data and facts with conviction and devotion
Surgery built on scientific advances of another
Better than listening to mother

Surgeons are made, not born. Development as a surgeon – scientist is not a business. It is a way of life. The family moved from grandmas home in upstate New York. First, an apartment in the Bronx, then to another apartment in Glen Oaks, Queens. Dad was a candy broker, Mom a full time homemaker. Summers were still spent at Grandma Essie's country farm. Previous schooling was at a rural school in Fleischmans. All grades were taught in one school room. Evidently, one size fits all. In the winter, three of us (brother Richard, sister Nancy) would walk down the hill to jump into the back of Charlie Barret's Ford pick-up for the ride to school. Winters were real tough.

The Catskills many trout streams were filled with native "Brookies." The water was clear, colorless and very cold from mountain water runoff. It tasted sweet. The trout were wily and very smart. They tasted just right when mom fried them. I was good with the traditional hook, line and sinker method. Somewhere along the way I adapted a hand to throat grabbing technique. Since the water was waist deep and the rocks slippery, this wasn't easy. Whenever this story is told, it's greeted with derision. It's a fish story and eyes roll upwards. My brother, sister and I laugh . . . we were there. This was the first manual dexterity test for this surgeon of the future. I was 12 years old.

Golf was self taught in Fleishmanns at the local Takanassee Hotel (now defunct) course. Played real good golf and was asked to give exhibitions before the hotel guests on Sunday. From caddying, to putting the caddies for cokes, to exhibiting my golf style, was self satisfying. The first tee was a par three, about 150 yards. There was no problem laying up next to the hole. My brother, Richard, would cash in for me by passing around the hat. The guests were quite generous in their donation to the local yokel. Money was hard to come by. And coke in the green bottle was a nickel then.

Baseball's a team sport. While living in Glen Oaks, there was a community baseball field across the street. This was my sanctuary . . . I spent all day, usually everyday at third base or pitching. Batting fourth and batting 400% in the PAL (Police Athletic League) ensured my participation in the local sandlot games. My pitching wasn't noteworthy. I still remember a left hand hitter crushing an inside fastball across the street and over the apartment buildings. It may still be in the clouds. Mother quashed any thoughts of a baseball career. She had other plans for me and baseball wasn't in my future.

Stanley Everett was my best friend. He married Toby. She was a girl friend of one date who rejected me. Stanley was brilliant, I was not. Stanley was in the top 5% of the graduating class in Jamaica High School. He was accepted to the University of Vermont – combined medical school program of seven years. I graduated in the top third of the class and had a dismal future. A memorable event were two amateur chemists making bromine in Stanley's garage at his house. His parents weren't home. We mixed the chemicals and thick clouds of reddish bromine gas filled the garage. We ran like hell into the street watching poisonous bromine billowing into the neighborhood. The wind was just right to dissipate the fumes. 911 was not a concept in those days. Stanley became a pediatrician and died of natural causes a few years ago. He will always be in my memory.

Queens College was my only option upon graduating Jamaica High. But fate was to decide my future.

A family trip to Montreal on Labor day, in 1956 allowed easy access to McGill Universities campus. Unbeknownst to my partents, I snuck off and obtained an application form. A little late perhaps to apply but Lucky Lew applied. A previous candidate decided to go elsewhere. McGill has geographic quota's; I was accepted and left a few days later on a Trans Canada flight, Giselle McKensy was on the flight. My parents were not amused. Played rugby on the intermediate team at McGill.

McGill was difficult but I graduated in 1960 with a Bachelor of Science degree. The honor of "distinction" for academic excellence was conferred. Was accepted at three Canadian Medical Schools and the Chicago Medical School. I suspect other U.S. medical schools confused the word "distinction" with "extinction."

Graduated the Chicago Medical School in June 1964. Passed the National Board exam. Interned at Jackson Memorial Hospital in Miami (U. of Miami's teaching hospital). Was promised the Ear Nose and Throat residency with successful completion of my rotating internship. Was on call 36 hrs/off 12 hrs. The pay was $300 a month. Received excellent training by Dr Sam Knight, chief Resident and Gordon Murley, in surgery. My good friend was Stanley Lewis, another abused intern. I remember Stanley because he was killed in Quang-tri in Nam. He joined the AIR-CAV. Even today it's painful for me to visit the "Wall."

Another memorable event was making rounds the first day. The first patient I saw was dead as a mackerel.

Though promised the residency in Ear Nose and Throat in Miami, I was rejected. My innocence came to an end. Medical politicians and administrators were never trusted again. I was accepted into the ENT residency program at the Medical College of Wisconsin in 1965. My four year residency included one year of general surgery. One memorable event was the hospital costume party. Charlie Aprahamian, Chief Resident in surgery, was Armenian. He wore a sweat shirt with the logo "SA" across the chest. "Super Armenian." He asked the ward secretary what the "SA" stood for. Her reply, "stupid ass." The ENT residency training under Doctor Roger Lehman and his staff was excellent. Besides full time staff and capable senior residents, Roger brought in out-of-town, Milwaukee doctors. Dr. Pat Shirra from Sheboygan. And senior staff from Rochester, Minnesota. I suppose the Mayo Clinic took pity on provincials. Fellow residents Roland Geretti, and wife Jan, lives in Arizona; and Gerald Schmitz, retired. We became board-certified and followed our destinies.

Doctor John Woods was chosen to head Plastic Surgery at the Mayo Clinic. He succeeded the famous surgeon, Doctor Ollie Beahrs. Not only a very capable surgeon and author, he was a musician and magician. He became Chairman of Plastic Surgery on professional merit. John was to follow in his footprints. Ollie could perform parotidectomy (removal of parotid gland) with facial nerve dissection (display of the seventh nerve branches in the face) in less than 30 minutes. John was of the same ilk, a parotidectomy in a half hour. Every surgeon I've spoken too, including Medical Society mavens say the same thing – impossible. Besides being a great surgeon, John introduced me to making rounds twice-a-day. This cockamamey idea was to be adopted by me. How many doctors make rounds twice a day. Being a resident, my question wasn't why? It was to do or die. Learned to hone my skills as a surgeon with John. He was to return to Mayo and became a lecturer, speaker and introduced many innovative techniques to the lexicon in breast surgery. He added a missionary zeal to his fame. My Veterans Administration notation in plastic surgery was memorable. I became well trained and fast.

After training at Veterans Administration hospital teaching program, I was enlisted into the U.S. Public Health Service from 1969-1971. The program was in the Navy, and we also covered the Coast Guard and Merchant Marine. Doctor Bernard March of John Hopkins headed up our Department. Bernie was an outstanding expert in throat diseases. Two Military Residents in ENT were trained by us. Ron Tinsley in Alaska, and Richard Carlson in Washington State graduated and passed their Boards. I passed my Boards in 1970 while in the service. My two year stint ended uneventfully with an honorable discharge.

My private practice in ENT started in Baltimore in 1971. Learning the politics of hospital staffs at various locations, I was invited to the staff of the old South Baltimore Hospitable. The newly renamed Harbor Hospital had a surgical training program and again, I trained residents. Spending 29 years on the staff until leaving for South Chester Medical Center because of illness. There were no emergency room requirements at the South Chester Medical Center. There were no problems with my patients in my many years service. Mixing academic pursuits with practice, I published two scientific papers. The first following the lecturing of Thane Cody, Chief in ENT at the Mayo Clinic, "Mastoidectomy for Chronic Serious Otitis Media," was published in the Journal of Laryngology and Otology in 1981. The other article, "Microscopic Analysis of the Mastoid Bone," was inspired by David Austin, Otologist. It was printed in the Laryngoscope in 1985. David was a Physician Scientist from the University of Illinois.

My use of the operating microscope in sinus surgery started in 1996 after a course at the University of Pittsburgh. Doctors Mark May and Barry Chaikin taught ethmoidectomies. They sent the buses at 7 A.M. to haul me to Shadyside Hospital for an all days teaching conference. The bus returned at 9 P.M. The schedule almost killed me. The course content was excellent and the new technology embraced.

My office practice specialized in the surgical treatment of obstructive sleep apnea, (OSA). My own experiences with OSA taught me lessons to be passed on to patients. The history and physical includes rigid or flexible nasal and throat endoscopy. The anatomy included the septum and nubbins of ethmoid fleshy tissues; or tonsils that fall forwards to reach the ankle. Flaccid and redundant throat tissue was VIP, at that time, as the cause of sleep apnea.

In my case, the computerized axial tomography (CAT) scan showed changes of infection or subtle changes in the anatomy of the sinus. OSA is associated with ethmoid disease. My CT scan showed small sinuses with questionable ethmoid sinusitis. At surgery, Doctor David Kennedy found polyps in my ethmoid sinus extending into the sphenoids. Changes in the ethmoid sinus CT always seem to be understated in OSA patients. Doctor David Austin suggested that changes in the volume of aerated mastoid (in this case – ethmoid) cells are decreased form chronic infection. The reduced volume is due to death cells of the mastoid system being replaced by bone. The deposition of calcium and other minerals demonstrates sclerosis. This can be seen on a lateral mastoid x-ray when the mastoid is measured. The ethmoid sinus has other overlapping boney structures. A 3-dimensional CT scan in the future will enable accurate volumetric studies.

The sleep studies ordered on my patients are gold-standard overnight studies. They are done at local hospitals sleep labs or University Centers (like U. of Pittsburgh). No sleep studies were read by me. Philipsburg hospital did not have a sleep lab.

One patient exhibited the findings of a megapolyp. The fleshy polyp protruded from inside the nose onto the upper lip. It hung, glistening like a garden slug. He tried to save money by "cutting" off the polyp at home using scissors. No nasal cortisone spray or injections would shrink it. An operation for a nose "cut" was carried out in the office. Local anesthesia was accomplished with use of epinephrine soaked cotton balls with cocaine flakes. A good feeling was also obtained. Blakesley instruments and surgical scissors with a headlight; and it was snip, snip. The removal of stalk and roots was the "Carrot operation." You can't find it in the scientific literature but this was the first American polyp-cut. This megapolyp is the first one since an intact fossilized Tyrannosaurus was discovered.

CHAPTER 8

Sleep Apnea a la Mode

Lewis Newberg is my name
Obstructive Sleep Apnea is my game
Conventional treatment over time
Perpetuates the sleep apnea crime
OSA has a progressive life cycle
Turning like spokes in a bicycle
Bells toll for me – later and forever
My experiments are quite clever

Defense against non-self foreign substances was to protect myself using cells and protein components. The evolution of a system to destroy foreign substances started in the prehistoric oceans. My allergy to allergens, like ragweed, is a hypersensitivity response to foreign molecules. Allergy is part of immunology. The scope and breadth of the science of immunology is more than a sneeze or wheeze.

Obstructive sleep apnea (OSA) is a disease of the immune system. My first sign was the usual obnoxious snoring. Accompanying symptoms included chronic mouth breathing and nasal blockage. Years of oral medications, steroids including cortisone nasal spray and allergy shots for desensitization didn't do the job. Collating the signs and symptoms in OSA was initiating a script never contemplated.

My concept of allergy as the only adaptive response to pollen was too narrow. There was the runny nose, itchy eyes and allergic salute. The concept of allergy within molecular biology causing my OSA was never considered. In any event, my supernatural powers as a young physician would ward off any serious disease. Habitual snoring was an annoyance. Chronic mouth breathing with nasal obstruction were accoutrements of allergy. The treatment of snoring for me and my patients – no problem. Under pressure from mother and wife to obtain a sleep study at South Baltimore General Hospital; this was done. I thought it would be a waste of time and money for me. OSA was becoming a problem in the 1980's; better safe than sorry. I was tired after a "good" or "not so good" nights sleep.

Stress from the pressures of my practice required frequent feedings in the "food" engine. Always on the run, exercise was a disease causing heart attacks in other young physicians. So what if my family made fun of my belly hanging over my belt to touch the knees. I was obese (fat), and successful. My son Ethan used the words "landing field" to describe the protrusion. It was time for a winter trip to Miami to join the other walrus's on the beach. We basked in the rays to obtain a beach ball sunburn. Bellies were great flotation aides. One could sleep floating and never drown. High blood pressure developed but who cared?

Hurricane winds at night from snoring were health risks. There were additional costs from structural damage to the house. The addition of laser and other "toys" for treating snoring advanced. Laser-assisted uvuloplasty (LAUP) was introduced by Doctor Joseph Krespi in New York. I underwent two LAUP procedures as an outpatient. My results were good temporary relief but a reduced snoring returned in 5-6 months. My breathing was also improved but drooling became an annoyance.

A sleep study was obtained showing mild sleep apnea. The number of the Respiratory Disease Index (RDI) was 10. Ten episodes per hour of absent and/or reduced breathing. This so-called upper air way resistance syndrome (UARS) was so mild in this period of time, it wasn't considered treatable. The main sign and symptom was excessive daytime sleepiness. A nap in the afternoon at the office on an exam table was monitored by my nurse. Falling off and breaking a leg is not the way to go.

Innate immunity was an old world creation. It lacked flexibility in responding to environmental changes. The adaptive modern immune system is a cellular mediated response. The humoral (antibody) defense are protective mechanisms starting in embryonic stem cells in the fetus. My immune system differed from Mom and Dad's. Their DNA is not alive, or capable of specifying all that I am. My immune system is more than the sum of its components. For example, my immune system differs in its life memory. Protection by a surveillance system of vigilance, Gort—type cells patrol my body. The recall of the immune response by repeated exposure of antigens separated by long periods of time is good. The environmental exposure to stimulation by antigens is covered from birth to death.

The development of the adaptic immune system was too late for run-around-Sue. She's the T-rex who asphyxiated from her sinus filters being plugged up. During a sneeze-roar she tripped and fell into a tar and rock pit. Forensics confirmed a mega-polyp death.

One can imagine a self organizing system of proteins coded by genes. The interconnections and relationships of cells, molecules, and subatomic particles are more than a genetic blueprint. The probability patterns of subatomic atoms suggest a relationship and interconnect originating with basic matter. Antigens tweaking B and T immune cells to send signals within the cytokine nanonetwork (CNN) leads to activation of the immune complexes.

The disturbing part of my sleep study result was a lowered oxygen level throughout the night. People without sleep apnea have mean oxygen levels 90-100 percent. Mine was reduced under 90% into the eighties. Sitting up at night to take a last "gasp" after absence of breathing was scary. Never awake enough to understand the danger; my life might be abbreviated. Only threw off the covers and was constantly tired.

The follow up to lowered blood oxygen were daily checks in the ICU using pulse oximetry. Observation of my low oxygen levels in the eighties must be faulty equipment. Reporting incorrect oxygen levels was checked by the nursing supervisor. The oximeters functioned perfectly. The only substandard measurement was my oxygen. Denial is a powerful and comfortable force.

My OSA progressively worsened in 1996. Sleep apnea was complicated by high blood pressure. Then, chest pain during surgery required my transport from the operating room to the emergency room. The signs and symptoms of a major heart attack were confirmed by the worst looking EKG I'd seen since medical school. I still remember the flashing blue and red lights of the ambulance on the trip to John Hopkins. It was a Friday night and the doors of the cath lab miraculously opened. Doctor Schaffer, my cardiologist from Harbor Hospital was on the staff of Hopkins. He performed the cath – and it was difficult. He was covered in sweat at the end of the procedure. An assisted device was placed into my heart after angioplasty, placed on the blood thinner heparin, followed by coumadin and other heart meds. A month later, I took the trip to Washington Hospital Center. Met with Doctor Garcia, Cardiac Surgeon extraordinary from the Philippines. My big enchilada was a three vessel coronary bypass operation. Dr. Garcia impressed me. He did thousands of cases. I noticed his thin spidery fingers were small. The incision would be small and there would be plenty of workroom. I gave permission to do "his thing."

After surgery, diabetes mellitus type 2 started. Oral hypoglycemics and insulin were needed. Today, as then, insulin requirements remain high due to insulin-resistant diabetes.

Psoriasis, an immune disease developed on my elbows. There is a family history of psoriasis. The surgery I developed cured two patients with psoriasis. Restless leg syndrome (jumpy legs) was present. This feeling of discomfort in my calves bothers me today. Congestive heart failure is an ongoing problem. My allergies expanded to include asthma. Allergy shots continue. To overcome OSA with signs and symptoms of the metabolic syndrome, a constant positive airway pressure (CPAP) machine is used. Survival from the living dead, to functional physician was accomplished. My discovery that OSA is a disease of molecular biology explains stigmata persisting in OSA.

My discoveries into the origin, cause and cure of OSA are based on reasoned thought. My personal experiences confirm OSA as a disease of molecular medicine. The uncovering of immune (mast) cells in ethmoid surgical tissue exposed the truth. The mast cell is an essential immune cell in OSA. And that the future of molecular medicine in curing disease is coming. The operation developed by me of combining sinus and throat surgery has cured many patients. This may be the greatest story I've ever told.

CHAPTER 9

Run-around-Sue
The Queen of Jurassic Park

Tyrannosaurus rex sniffed the breeze
Largest lizard to sneeze and wheeze
Standing on hind legs was complex
Fossilized arms clutching kleenex
Modern introduction to immunity
A product of Rexie's community
The mast cell didn't arise from the void
It's a product of the ethmoid

T-rex was the most terrible, ill tempered lizard in the age of nasty meat eating reptiles. It had 12 inch teeth to eat you better. I suspect it was not scavenging for carrion.

Death of T-rex is the subject of speculation. Antigenic and dust overload in the atmosphere blocked Reggies nose and made him ill. Breathing became labored from pollens of the trees and grasses striking the ethmoid nasal lining. Innate immunity would provide a protective shield against large pollens. This was analogous to a shower curtain in the bathtub. Shower droplets cannot penetrate the plastic. The smaller molecular particles would pass through the netting into the deeper ethmoid cells and tissues. They would trigger an immune adaptive response to allergens. Poor Sue! The immune system was under development. The final construction was never witnessed. Smaller subatomic particles entering Rexie's lungs caused spasms in the tissues and wheezing. The adaptive response related to future gene splicing and rearrangement only produced the slobber gene. Rexie was a chronic mouth breather with nasal blockage and asthma. The famous "sneeze-roar" is vintage Rexie. The slobber and bad breath were tip offs to an inadequate immune system. The fossil demonstrates Rexie with a box of Kleenex.

The finding of a complete fossilized T-rex in South Dakota (call me Sue) documented an immune system under construction. Sue was under attack of killer insects and antigens. There as a humongous nasal polyp blocking the left nostril. Unfortunately, a large cockroach was wedged in the right side and started fluttering it's wings. The sneeze-roar of Sue, honking of Hadrosaurs and buzzing of insects of insects was the Cretaceous music of the night. Labored breathing and shortness of breath required a 911 call. But it was too late. Sue fell into a tar pit and was buried in rock and sand for 65 million years. Sue had a rudimentary yet distinct ethmoid sinus. Only one cavity on each side – the passage of time had destroyed the thin egg-thick ethmoid cellular system. There were red cells found and bony canals to support small nerves and vessels to the sinus. The organ of smell adjacent to the ethmoid sinus was large. Rexie could smell well until allergies and polyps struck. Run-around-Sue, the extinct Cretaceous T-rex now resides in a private suite on Lake Shore Drive, Chicago.

65 million years ago, a meteorite smashed into the Yucatan in Mexico. The Chicxulub crater is a study in atmospheric extinction of many species. Hitting with the force of 2 thousand atom bombs, dust particles reached into the atmosphere for six months. Dust, ash and steam turned light into day and photosynthesis stopped. The crater is not much of a tourist attraction. Looking into a big hole in the ground doesn't do it for most people. This extinctive explosion introduced new species. The age of the kosher chicken and mammals began.

CHAPTER 10

Attack of the Killer Roach

Prehistoric cockroaches ate volcanic ash
The modern roach eats trash
A killer roach attack
Provides a lot of allergy extract

The oldest pre-historic insect contributing body parts for my allergy extracts was the cockroach. Reaching land from the sea, Roachie occupied a crevice in volcanic rock. His meal was basic ash. He flourished in the Permian period and he grew big—real big. The earlier Devonian roach walked onto land 400 million years ago. Borne with three teeth, one wing and a dysfunctional egg laying depositor that touched the ground. Roach enemies could follow the egg trail. The wings evolved into two real air beaters that sounded like cicada song. The full set of teeth allowed a better well rounded diet. The oviduct retracted into her body and reproduction was protected. The Permian-Triassic extinctive event did not destroy this king of the pre-historic bugs. Roachie survived as an immutable, tough as nails, no nonsense creep.

The exponential growth of the cockroach was to reach the zenith in Jurassic park. He was hardy, fat and resourceful. He could fast for a month without food. He developed the trick of crawling onto Tyrannosaurus Rex's belly. His craving for food was satisfied by pieces of meat or bone. One major antic was the propensity to climb from Rexies belly up a nostril. Nasal blockage and fluttering wings drove Rexie crazy.

Hundred's of million years later they met my family. The dried out skeletons of cockroaches were still airborne particles that caused allergies. But they adapted to modern culture. Roach and clip became synonymous. No longer considered a predatory scavenger, they're our buddies. I don't think so. Roach clips are common utensils found in vacations. Ask for a hemostat during surgery; "pass the clip." This sophisticated use of the "roach clip" includes designer pins in Neiman-Marcus. Complete inventories of roach clips are in upscale head shops.

Leasing timeshare in Miami Beach is big business. Roaches love Jewish garbage in the winter. Bagels, cakes and condiments are prime sources of roach haute cuisine. Jewish garbage brings premium lease arrangements. Roachie, a big shot executive, was the ultimate proselytizing timeshare specialist. Misrepresentation as a "survivor" of extinction, he appealed mother's attempt to squish him with her shoe. His mantra "a good roach is a clean roach." Mother recognized him as a Paleozoic liar.

My family's rejection of roaches signaled the beginning of the "Bagel" war. It would reach a fever pitch. The battlefield was a space between the sink and fridge. Equivalent in viciousness to the Battle of Thermopyle, the Charge of the Light Brigade, or the Sugar Ray Leonard-Marvelous Marvin Hagler fight, no quarter was given, none asked. This battle – royale ended when mother knocked out this dysfunctional roacheroo with a heavy chicken pot to the head. With the clout of an axe roachie went down and out for the count. At the count of one, the coupe-de-grace was administered, squishing Roachie with her heel. Mom's comment summed up the situation well, "A good roach is a dead roach."

News of the "kitchen roach massacre" in Miami Beach spread quickly and widely on the Internet. The brotherhood of Roach species in Florida are the Palmetto bugs. Retribution would be swift and noisy. A contract from prehistoric relatives was arranged. Big bucks passed hands. This band of "immortal" roaches would be led by "Vinnie the Hood."

The palmetto bus motored up Florida State Highway 826, the Palmetto expressway to the Collins Avenue exit. A frontal, daylight airborne assault was planned. The assault was obvious because of cicada-like noises from their wings. It was no surprise to Mom and Dad. They waited at my brother Richards home in Golden Beach for the attack. Mom's instincts and techniques were a combination of raptor and T-rex slash and rip moves. After the slaughter, Mom nonchalantly said "they came in the same old way, and were dispatched of in the same old way." No roach approached our home again. To this day, roaches scatter for cover in bright light. Today sneaky cockroaches are scavengers and walk from kitchen to bedroom at night. A short jump, and then it's just a skip to the pillow. If you hear scratching in the pillow at night, get up and run.

CHAPTER 11

The Shtick of Mighty Mite

Trilobites crawled from the seas
Evolving into dust mites was the key
Eight hairy legs and blind
Eating skin scales of human kind
Mighty mite developed the first sex hormone
It was the pungent fecal pheromone
Fecal desiccated dust mites up the nose
Required removal with a flexible hose
The fate of horny dust mites
Is repeated in countless hypersensitivity flights
Home are carpets, mattresses and bedding
Gifts of a life time wedding
The desiccated mite leaves airborne fecal pellets, saliva and shells
Allergy shots work quite well!

Dust mites are associated with house dust. The dust mite came from the sea onto land in the Permian period 250 million years ago. This is the walking trilobite that evolved 8 legs. They live on skin scales in the bedding. They are always thirsty for a drink of water through their leg joints. It's the humidity of ones skin sweat that furnishes moisture. This prehistoric arthropodic fish produces the strongest immune response of all the inhalant antigens. Skin testing and shots will bring this allergen under control. Even with dry conditions in mattresses, it takes months for mites to croak or antigen levels to fall. My allergy extracts for skin testing contain European and American dust mite antigens.

Species come; species go. If there is no fossil evidence proving the existence between two species, a Lazarus taxus is witness to resurrection of the species. Purification of dust mite allergens shows a glycoprotein. Positive skin reactions are frequent and intense.

The evolution of the dust mite extended from the Jurassic period into the Cretaceous period of reptiles. The dust mite took on the appearance of a mole. Large hairy front legs for pulling his body along the fecal trail. Eight legs clawed their way from Tyrannosaurus Rex's belly into his nose. With the hardness of cuticle, these legs were made for walking; up your nose. The first "trail" of pheromones allowed his schmageggi brothers to follow the scent to paradise ranch. The pheromones were the first sign of a complex protein hormone. The haute cuisine of dust mites was the ethmoid filet mignon. The best cuts of meat were found in Area 51 where epithelial cells were lined in tandem. Soft, succulent ethmoid cells extended to the corral at the "Ranch."

We have little protection from a dust mite attack. Dust mites were fierce and ferocious warriors assaulting the thin mucus line covering the ethmoid cells. This gossamer layer could only collect the atmospheric antigens of airborne desiccated dust mite shells, feces and saliva. The whole mucus and epithelial layer resembles mosquito netting. The large fragments that were caught could be expressed in a booger. The smaller particles passed through the filter to the deeper ethmoid tissues. All kinds of havoc in Rexie's nose made him sick.

Modern day dust mites die and become airborne antigens. They live off skin flakes when you sleep. Occasionally, a family of dust mites will regress to their ancestry.

The trek from bedding is a short space. Dust mites are too small to be seen with the naked eye. A creepy-crawling feeling in your nose that awakes you is cause for alarm. Sit up, blow your nose, and dial 911. Tell the operator "Booger alert." This is a bona-fide emergency requiring a vacuum cleaner up the nose—with a flexible hose.

CHAPTER 12

The Cotillion Ball
Or
Cells of the Immune System

I am a Yankee Doodle Cell
This is my story to tell
Tissue mast cells
Produce hormones from hell
Hormones are stored in the Golgi
This is not baloney!
Round and round the witches brew
Boiling a supernatural stew

The city is New York. The setting is the ballroom in the refurbished Trump Towers. A masquerade ball was followed by the cotillion march up Fifth Avenue. The winner is crowned "Queen of the Night." Cinderella's horse-drawn carriage parades past Bergdorf Goodman stopping at Tiffany's. The first prize is all you can pick and mix among the gold baubles. It's fill the golden wheelbarrow in 30 seconds. Then it's on to 5th and 34th for an exclusive and private tour of the Garment District. This Ball is the yearly coming out party for the young and beautiful white cells.

A Masquerade Ball preceded the formal debutante march to the dais. Paris Hilton greeted guests from a bubble bath on the stage. Her new bath oil derived from a natural hormone, an isomer of Love Potion #9. This hormone is a derivative of the tissue mast cell. To emphasize the importance, she stunned the crowd rising from the bath water in her birthday suit. Yes, kitch is alive and functioning well in New York.

Blood basophils have a multi-headed nucleus with large pink cytoplasmic granules. She resembled a sequin covered gown without any makeup. The head rotates like a turret on a Tiger Tank. The red polka dots suggested a permanent case of measles. When I was in medical school, the conventional wisdom was that the blood basophil changed into a tissue mast cell. We know that the mast cell has one head, and the structural scaffolding is different. The production of the allergic antibody IgE and cytokines are miniscule in blood basophils. The release of histamine pales in comparison to mast cells. She made the yearly trek to the cotillion ball—she never won – too pink.

The eosinophil, another beautiful immune cell, was last years winner. Her output of histamine was up, but cytokines production was flat. Though a past winner, she was scandalized by a lack of propriety. Her La Perla underwear was transparent. She overcame her year-long embarrassment. To bolster her courage, she resorted to a snort of the white powder.

Mona, the blood monocyte, sprang forth from the bone marrow stem cell. She had a large bilobed nucleus described as a "bubble head." She had foamy holes in her brain and was considered slow on the uptake (if you get my drift!) Her big swim in blood ended with migration into sinus tissues. She had developed a curved nucleus and her physical form changed. She became a hippie. This free thinker wore a tasteless, but colorful thong swimwear. This was a metallic green rhinestone bikini: with a wrap around toga. This twenty foot sash was haute couture. Lots of fake Fortunoff jewelry inscribed with "made in France." No Walmart label "made in China." The Ros Hammerson sandals completed the ensemble

The metamorphosis from Mona to a macrophage paralleled the egg—pollywog—frogette—frog's changes. The macrophage has all kinds of amebic movements and shapes. The macrophage is one ugly looking brute. It has a special relationship with T lymph's. Derived from a species of shape shifters, it has the dexterity to bob, weave and undulate around and through surrounding ethmoid cells. This dance of life parallels rope-a-dope moves under the scanning electron microscope; they appear as kraken. Their resemblance to garden slugs secreting mucous trails and gliding from one area to another was uncanny.

Her innovative fashion statement was wearing a tutu with tank top and ballet shoes. This creature shocked the fashion writers. The jewel of her garb was an imitation "wicked witch of the west" costume. One writer quipped she should wear a broom! Then an artificial broom was shoved up her rump. One influential writer said "I don't believe what I'm seeing." Another, "what a pig." A positive comment (by her mother) "what brilliance, imagination and precision."

The Mast cell, known among friends and jealous foes as Nasty Masty. She's a reddish purple, metachromatic cell, borne into a dysfunctional bone marrow matrix. She has difficulty categorizing herself as a health car giver. She has many functions but is no friend of humanity. Possessing a single nucleus with seeds of purple granules, she has production facilities for the machinery to make complex proteins. Under the electron microscope, the granules resemble peppercorns.

Her problem was overeating. She ate lots of organelles derived from blintzes. The digestive enzymes in the organelles contained rich yogurts. The mast cell got bigger and bigger. She resembled an overripe hemorrhoid. At the ball, she wore an Oscar De La Renta designer dress with Manola Blahnik pumps. Very sheik! At the masquerade ball, Nasty was able to camouflage the purple granules containing biochemical mediators. The mediators contain large amounts of histamine and are associated with acute hypersensitive immune responses. Whether bee-stings or ragweed antigen, the immediate response could be overwhelming and permanent. The Ig E antibody – mast cell activation may initiate this cathartic cleaning. The acute phase of release of cytokine mediators may be this cellular bulemia.

The activation of the mast cell triggers the release of biochemical mediators. The histamine and heparin play major roles in the acute hypersensitivity reactions. With repeated exposure to the same antigen, the response may be shorter. Instead of a chronic release of mediators taking 2-3 days, it may elicit an acute reaction. A "leaky mast cell" for release of mediators from guar gum (plant) antigen may accelerate. Occupation exposure may induce acute OSA.

Under the influence of the environment, the mast cell has seen, and responded to new signaling messages. There has been an increase number of cytokines from processing of sushi antigens. Cytokines guide and modulate the manufacturing sequences to produce complex neuropeptides. These neuropeptides were originally identified as Brand X with the blueprint of a gene; the Brand X can be separated into hormones. The first hormone was the pheromone. This attracted mates. Then a new neuropeptide was constructed in the machinery in a mast cell. The Garment District in New York City would learn these old world techniques and technology to their advantage. And a derivative of the newest hormone – Love Potion #9 – caught Paris Hiltons smell buds. She was to sign a licensing agreement for this bath oil perfume.

The commercial contract between Paris and Nasty Masty was looked upon favorably. The arrangement was a solicitation. The Cotillion Ball was to terminate in the debutante march to the dais. This was a show stopper. Nasty would advertise; anything to win.

She celebrated her victory with an advertising blitz beginning with a slide-show of her latest electron microscopy photos. She pointed out structures resembling multiple torahs. Within the scroll were caricatures of Monte Cristo cigars. The labels said "made in Israel."

The neuropeptide, Neurotrophic Growth Hormone (NGH) has been plagued by manufacturing glitches. Complex cells are committed to a programmed cell death in response to internal signals. It can sense its useful life is over. Apototic death is a bummer.

NTG is stored in the Golgi apparatus. Then it's excreted through a Johnny Flusher into the blood for the trip to distant tissues. The complex hormones are quality controlled proteins. They must be a model molecules. Charlie tuna didn't make the cut-off; Charlie is and will always be a loser.

CHAPTER 13

The Dynamic Duo

Those magnificent B and T lymphocytes
Two shining bright lights
Cells and plasma proteins mount the defenses
Destroying antigens with immune responses
Lymphocytes are the only cells to rearrange genes
Providing bouillabaisse at the cellular scene
Adaptic immunity is more than chromosomes
It's an environmentally driven genome
Lymphocytes can talk, the talk!
Now they walk, the walk!

The big-bang started the big show 13 billion years ago (bya). Two electrons collided in the vacuum of space. The universe became a finite entity. The debris of rocks, dust particles, gases and cosmic rays would form an ever expanding universe.

Proteins were produced in the first unicellular life forms of bacteria and fungi. Planet Earth was a molten mass of gases, hydrogen and helium. Cooling of the earth and the bombardment of earth with space debris contained other elements consisting of carbon, nitrogen, sulfur and a host of others we are carbon based units and atmospheric gene fragments were incorporated into cells. DNA and chromosomes were identified. A plasma membrane developed to cover the cell providing separation of the cell from the environment. It turned out as a bi-layer fat sandwich of complex proteins, the phospholipids. This interface between the living interior of the cell, and non-living exterior is regulated by the movement of molecules in and out of the cell.

Every cell in our body contains the information necessary to specify our physical structure. The information is the genome, written in DNA as a string of 3 billion letters that consist of an alphabet of only four bases: A-adenine, T-thymine, C-cytosine, and G-guanine. The gene is a piece of DNA that carries permanent information. The DNA is like a curved parallel ladder; this is the scaffolding or backbone of the DNA helix. The rungs of the ladder are 3 billion base pairs as cross-ties.

God's chosen cell for an innate and adaptable immune system is the lymphocyte. This is the linchpin of the immune system. They're foetal in development and develop the complex proteins necessary to differentiate into mature forms. These "naïve" lymphocytes never encounter a foreign antigen until they are schooled and taught their proper functions. They develop the specificity and distinctness toward antigens they never met. Their maturity before release is by surface proteins that are graded on cluster of Differentiation (CD) markers. Precursors of B-lymphocytes (B-cells) mature in the bone marrow (the Bursa of Flavius). T-lymphocytes attain maturity in the thymus gland. The mature lymphocytes are released into the sinus tissues. They are attracted to nasal inflammation.

Our host defense system of immunity protects us from foreign chemical or antigen substances. The lymphocyte is the lead cell to destroy non-self foreign bodies. Allergy is the study and treatment of human hypersensitivity reactions producing inappropriate immune responses.

The molecular biology of lymphocytes consists of heavy and light chain molecules. The making of the immunoglobulin molecule (Ig G) requires a number of alternative genes to combine into a single complete protein molecule. The B lymphocyte (Bursa of Fabricus) is an adaptive humoral response to produce antibodies. The code for the heavy chains is on chromosome 14, those for light chains on chromosomes 2 and 22. Twenty-three chromosomes, 20,000 genes and billions of base pairs lead to diversity in the immune system.

The naïve lymphocyte encountering a lymphocyte that has processed an antigen of distinct and specific function, can produce clones. They have immune memory to respond quickly, and with greater intensity to repeated antigen exposure. The lymphocyte has surveillance technique to respond. An inappropriate immune response can lead to tissue injury and death of a cell.

The interconnections between atoms and molecules, cytokines and the innate and adaptive immune systems allows for probabilities and probability patterns to activate an immune complex. A generous macromolecule, like a flounder caught in the wind, would stretch the netting. The cytokine nanonetwork (CNN) has a global pattern. The surface layer of innate immunity would allow smaller antigens to contact the ethmoid epithelial layer. The adaptive response of B and T lymphocytes influence the production of complex neuropeptides. Subatomic particles may bypass the entire immune complex and go directly to the lungs. Asthmas is particularly responsive to subatomic particles.

Lymphocytes appear rather common. They are plain Janes. A simple light grey cell, an average sized one-headed nucleus led to disqualification from the Cotillion Ball. If you've seen one lymphocyte, you've seen them all. They are the one and only cell in our body to rearrange its genes from environmental clues. The function of our immune system depends on exposure to antigens.

Lymphocytes rearrange their genome as they differentiate from foetal or bone marrow stem cell to mature B or T cell.

The B lymphocyte is an immunoglobulin molecule composed of four complex proteins. Two heavy and two light chains. The rearranged genes allow DNA to rearrange its genes into messenger RNA (mRNA). The immunoglobulin G type can undergo isotope switching from IgG to Ig E antibodies. This Ig E antibody anchors itself to a mast cell in the deeper ethmoid tissues. The plasma cell of the bone marrow flows in the blood. It provides a back up source of Ig E antibody. The plasma cell is as common as the lymphocyte in the eyes of judges in the Cotillion Ball.

The molecular biology of T cells is similar to B cells except the proteins produced in the rearrangement must stay as surface receptor molecules. These four proteins simulated onion on a bialy. The mature T cell has skin resembling early wrinkles. A change in membrane lining would require Botox, no artificial enhancers were allowed in the application for the Ball. Where as an antigen binds directly with an Ig E antibody mast cell complex, the receptor molecule on a T cell acts indirectly with foreign antigen.

A new application was introduced. DNA rearranging its genes while passing through the nuclear membrane to mRNA was the "tschotske" cell. The cell developed the cytokines to digest kosher chickens. This "tschotske" cell could expel waste at a prodigious rate; like lasix.

The mRNA is intimately involved in complex protein synthesis. The rough endoplasmic reticulum's with little buttons of ribosome's on their surface have manufacturing capability. The assembly of complex proteins is destined for the Golgi apparatus for storage and transport to distant tissue sites.

Ig E is also produced in the plasma cell, an immune cell from bone marrow. A clone of Ig E antibody molecules is assured. The Ig E antibody anchors to a mast cell lying near sinus tissues. Light and heavy chains sprout from the surface mast cell with the hydra-like claws, seeking to capture a whole kosher chicken or sushi antigen. The Ig E mast cell complex is activated by an antigen when the key fits into the lock. The release of biochemical mediators by this sushi trigger, are large amounts of histamine and lesser quantities of heparin. The breakdown of arachidonic acid releases chemical mediators of the lipoxygenase pathway and the release of leukotriene (LT4). This releases the mucous of sinus tissues and contributes to cellular injury.

One ancillary discovery of importance: B and T cells release separate molecules, from whole antigens or fragments respectively. The Chinese menu has its origin in listing choices of dishes; one from column A and two from column B., this catalyst also suggested the everyday tools of Chinese food; chopsticks.

The adaptic immunity of B cells, so-called humoral immunity, involves antibody Ig E. The hydra-like arms from the light chains capture a whole antigen. Capturing a whole kosher chicken in the claws of the light and heavy chains is the B cell way.

T cells are adaptic cell mediated fragments of proteins involving surface proteins. These peptide or lipoprotein fragments are chicken giblets. Macrophages or the new viscous gank cells can rip apart meat.

The bar bell weight lifter gets a tutorial in T cell recognition. A T cell attaches to a peptide bar which is fixed to an antigen presenting cell (APC). The peptide bar comes into contact with the T cell and APC. The bar is a Nathans hot dog. The hot dog bun is a T cell receptor (TCR) and a major histocompatiblitiy complex MHC). The biological basis for antigen recognition is in the context of MHC molecules is to distinguish self from non-self. This T cell complex is surrounded by a CD4 surface protein on one side, and a super antigen on the other. They appear like booster rockets. Activation of the complex is by a "pickle-tickle." Helper T cells function for the B cells, and production and release of cytokines like tumor necrosis factor (TNF) and interferon. The immune response is dependent on the T cell complex activation. Carbohydrate fragments of an Oreo cookie, or even a Fig Newton, may accomplish T cell activation when a macrophage shatters a cookie.

The sushi antigen provides a maximal immunological response of a new antigen. This antigen may be wrapped around the T complex as a super antigen or a CD4 protein. The addition of a low molecular weight hapten is not potent except when linked to a large carrier protein. Duration of exposure and number of lymphocytes in the vicinity are important factors, and may represent some import in the strength of the autoimmune response.

The lymphocyte never met an antigen it didn't want to eat. Processing of sushi antigen to mince meat provides signals to the bone marrow and other immune cells. The T lymphocytes are becoming more active. Ferocious gank cells may replace macrophages one day.

The signals to the mast cell for the production of complex neuropeptides seem to be increasing. Neurotrophin Growth Hormone (NGH) is taking an increased cause in the origin and cause of OSA.

CHAPTER 14

The Pollen Wars
and
The Sushi Antigen

Ancient oceans filled by rain
Atmospheres choked with clouds of pollen grain
Innate immunity is the prehistoric protective defense
Plasma protein complement and mucous are a pretense
The modern immune system evolved an adaptive stance
Adaptive immunity is the way for mankind to advance
Cytokine nanonetwork (CNN) stretches to cover our tuckus
Pollens croak in ethmoid mucous
Crossing the River Styx between heaven and hell
Charon ferries her cargo; just ring the bell!
Sushi antigens are different sizes and shapes
Complex 3-D special configurations and weights
Adaptic immunity prevents Run-around-Sue's crime
It's development took eons of time
Previous extinctive events of ice ages and meteors
We can witness Pollen Wars on tour!

Today, Planet Earth is witness to temperate climates with dry atmospheric conditions. Past global warming had led to exuberant growths of stamens, anthers, and pollen sac's. The overabundance of pollens gave flowering trees, plants, weeds, and grasses the opportunity to dominate nature. The world was a machine and a plot was hatched to dominate the world: They needed growing room. This mechanistic and simple view would acknowledge that some questions in life will remain a mystery.

The gunfight at the OK Corral pitted Marshall Earp and his brothers with Doctor Holliday representing law and order. Big Nose Kate, Doc's girlfriend, was the lookout. The Clantons and other cowboys were rustlers. The battle was a deadly shootout at the OK Corral. Law and order was the winner over open banditry. The death of the Clantons prevented rustling. Another famous Marshall, "Wild Bill" Hickok, was shot in the head from behind in a saloon in Deadwood Gulch, in the Black Hills in the Dakota territories. Crooked Nose McCall was the villain; Bill was gunned down at poker with the Dead Mans Hand, 2 pairs of aces and eights. The status quo was enforced by violence.

Unbeknownst to all, the understanding of life in an expanding world fell to the Pollen Industrial Complex.

The Pollen Industrial Complex Generals were familiar with attacking fixed fortifications. The Maginot Line in France, with its parallel and opposite Siegfried lines, was studied. These were monuments to the stupidity of mankind. Of course, the pollens weren't graduates of Cal Tech. Killer roach and dust mite antigens would lead the dive bombing assault on the outer defenses. Pollen casualties would be high. Caesar crossing the Rubicon to invade Gaul turned the river red. Dead soldiers floated by. Another blood bath was planned.

The primary attack would be an amphibious assault into the outer mucous layer and crossing the River Styx which was filled with plasma protein complement. This river formed the boundary between the nasal air cavity and the building blocks of the sinus cavity. The River Styx was a prehistoric defense against large molecules of the pollen kind. The live pollens would be transported by tugboat and ferry across the river by Charon.

River Styx abutted bricks of the epithelial layer. The sinus defenses were considerable and were stretched to the maximum. Adaptic humoral immunity (antibodies) and cell mediated immunity (T cells) awaited the pollen invasion. The defense cells of macrophages, lymphocytes and glycoprotein modulators and facilitators had almost 100 million years to evolve. They were initially anchored by mighty Achilles. Then it was "Dirty Harry" of "make my day." A future back up cell of immune memory and surveillance was a Gort-type of networking. The war cry of "klatto barada nikto" was being taught. In the future, this simple statement would trigger panic in the attackers. My mother may have known this command. She used it effectively on my brother and me.

A divisionary attack of goldenrod pollen was decided. Goldenrod was mistaken for ragweed pollen. Goldenrod has heavy, wet, sticky pollen with a pungent, sweet nauseating smell. It was a poor choice to transfer across the Styx as its constituency was insects. There was the consistency of hearty barley soup. There was a great loss of life before the attack took place. Goldenrod died by drowning. Charon had no choice but to transfer the dead and dying to the far side of the river. Charon cleaned up from the additional revenue. He was well known for taking bribes for safe passage.

The final battle was as disastrous as "The Charge of the Light Brigade." Was there a pollen grain dismayed? No way! There were macrophages to the right of them, B and T lymphocytes to left of them. Ganks, cytokines, future Gorts, and plasma proteins made mincemeat of them. Whole pollen grains were seized by antibodies. Fragment of protein and lipoprotein were processed by T lymphocytes. They fought well but very few returned from hell.

The nasal inflammatory response was world-wide. This prelude to world domination was a fiasco. But who knew? Only the Shadow knows! He hung deep in the ethmoid tissues processing the abundance of fresh meat.

The extinctive events to obliterate all living organisms started 4 ½ billion years ago when hydrogen and helium were the only elements of Earth. Since we are carbon based units, the carbon was added from other planets in space dust. Snippets of prehistoric DNA with the effects of gravity and time-space dimensions allowed a protective immune system to develop. Unicellular life joined other cells to produce multi cellular complex life with specialized functions. Immunity describes the functions of early host defense. The early primitive host defense system gave protection against chemicals an foreign substances. Viruses, fungi and bacteria have evolved independent systems for self preservation.

The B cell receptor of the "Bursa of Flavius" was derived from South Sea kosher chickens swimming for their lives. T cell receptors are abundant. When activated, T cells allow the immune functioning of B cells (antibodies).

Prototaxites, the humongous fungus of the upper Devonian Period survives today. A living fossil, its mycelia and hyphae disburse spore and little button mushrooms are alive and well. They are the size of large trees and are living fossils. Innate immunity may have saved them from the bacteriaphages and viruses.

Evolution was slow. T-rex fossils showed the early development of the ethmoid sinus and blood cells.

The various pollens causing allergies would be supplemented by plant antigens. Guar gum and hay fever not only caused sniffles, but OSA and asthma. This generic response would be immediate. Pollens had old fashioned values of "love and marriage go together like the horse and carriage." The Farmers Almanac supplanted teachings from the bible. It took on the religious symbolism. The seed catalogue had mystical religious overtones. Pollen grains discussed possibility of a religious war. Ragweed pollen clans were now armed with over 38 different proteins on the surface. All are highly allergic and support in the mucous layer attracted more pollens. Smaller subatomic particles could bypass the lung and go directly into the lungs causing asthma. The extinctive events in prehistoric times were usually environmental. Ice ages, meteors, and volcanic eruptions skewed the development of life on Earth.

Airborne antigens or foreign substances were the first travelers into the atmosphere. These were the lightweight bacteria, fungi and viruses. They caused immune responses in animals and T-rex. Basic sizes and shapes of pollens became more complex due to volcanic dust. A dust bowl Earth policy was developing into the extinctive kind. The rapid changes in the environment are suggesting a polluted poisoned planet. The new designer antigens affected the genes. OSA and the autoimmune disease are on a roll.

My clinical practice changed dramatically from 1980 onwards. There was an exponential increase in OSA cases. I suspect there is a concomitant rise in cases of asthma, diabetes, and obesity. The usual protein lore of an antigen may change. Spines on the surface of ragweed hide little furrows and grooves for special foreign antigens. Perhaps contaminants or pollutants change the spatial configuration. These subatomic particles are haptens. The comparison to sushi is like an add-on of a condiment. Fish eggs or sesame seeds on the surface can change the character of an antigen. This might be a Newberg "porcupine roll." A new airborne sushi antigen was borne.

The sushi antigen finesses the oldies but goodies. The new super-duper antigen has the ability to change the genome. The severe effects of the changes in genes alter the clinical expression. The sushi antigen penetrated into the deeper ethmoid tissues. Sushi antigens would be processed by immune cells, and signals sent to the bone marrow. Signals from the new sushi antigens would meet macrophages, lymphocytes and natural ganks. The four proteins, 2 light and 2 heavy chains are Ig E components. They resemble kraken with jaws that bite and claws that catch the sushi family. Jumping ge hosifat, the sushi antigen, antibody E, and mast cell, line up in tandem. They have formed a Qin Terra Cotta Army held in perfect formation by loosely bound ligands. These ligands are like rubber bands; they are reversible when the mast cell population is decimated by my operation. A signal passes from the antigen down the assembly with Ig E and mast cell. It's like a pickle tickle. The activation is not an explosion, but a belch. Biochemical mediators are released from the mast cell. There's action in the fancy pin ball machine tonight! Come light my fire!

The pollen wars led to changes in the color of nasal polyps. The dying and dead pollens matched the coal dust in miner's lungs. Red for infectious and inflamed tissues in the river. Glistening, opaque, green pea-like grapes were associated with allergies.

The development of immune gene snippets to evolve into the modern adaptive system may have started from plasmids in the atmosphere. Independent DNA molecules would be capable of independent replication. It might be circular and single or double stranded DNA to RNA. It may rearrange genes from chromosomes first this way, than the other. But it's the DNA and RNA that determines our well-being. Our genome depends on the genes, and the environment. And the all seeing, all powerful lymphocyte that rearranges genes adds immune protection into the future.

The cellular immunity of T-cells, or the antibodies produced by B cells, contains the same four complex proteins. The T cell fragments are presented to antigen producing cells and processed internally. The antibodies proteins are processed anchored to a mast cell. The light and heavy chains are identical but process antigen distinctly and separately. The T cell is the modulator for B cell activity.

The sushi antigens, using signals processed by B and T lymphocytes promote the synthesis of new hormones. The signals are the result of the ambush at the OK Corral. Wyatt would be proud of the removal of antigen. He would be disappointed with the growth of new hormones of the mast cell kind. Increasingly complex neuroproteins are the stuff autoimmune diseases are made of.

There is an increase of OSA during the allergy season. The finding of the by-products of mast cell activity in patients with OSA was interesting. Nasal inflammation showed an increase in biochemical mediators in the nose and urine. My findings of mast cells in surgical material of the ethmoid sinus correlate well with others. Guar gum, a plant antigen from shrubs (legumes) that are used in the ice cream and dog food industries, shows observable evidence of allergy and OSA. Documentation showed the correlation of an occupational plant antigen and OSA. Insuffilation of guar gum dust into an inhalant chamber triggered acute OSA. Removal of the employee from the guar gum allowed OSA to disappear. Here, as in the cases I've operated upon, OSA is reversible. And the ligands, or chemical bonds I rail about have the strength and staying power of rubber bands. The destruction of the myelin covering sheath in multiple sclerosis is irreversible; function may be lost forever.

Also the production of cytokines from lipooxygenase pathways in the break down of arachidonic acid. These include the leukotrienes (notably LT4) which have specific effects on the ethmoid cells. Mast cells are the gateway to OSA.

The mast cell has many products that cause harm. The DNA from the mast cell nucleus has transferred genetic material into the cell via messenger RNA to the site of protein synthesis. Ribosome's, little box cars are attached to the engine adjoining a railroad line. They enter the rough-looking surface tubules through the nuclear lining. Amino acids are turned into complex proteins. The Golgi is the final stage in production for the neuropeptides neurotrophin. This neurotrophic growth hormone (NTG) crosses Captain Kirk's neutral zone. This compares to our blood brain barrier (BBB). The receptor site sits on the membrane of a target neuron. This neurotransmitter is bound to the receptor and translates receptor occupation into electrical or chemical responses.

CHAPTER 15

Neurotoxins and Cytokine Storm

This is my story, sad but true
People with untreated sleep apnea have no clue
The mast cells neurotrophin affects neural wiring,
This hormone causes neural misfirings
Apneas and hypopneas affect sleep
Families and patients do weep
Reggie White and Momma Cass too
Its sudden death for these two

Cytokines are signaling proteins that control cells. They can signal T cells and macrophages to the site of inflammation. They modulate production of these cells, stimulating them to produce more cytokines. But if the immune system encounters a new and highly pathogenic invader, say a virus, uncontrollable cytokine storms occur in various tissues. Many cytokines are raised in the perfect storm. Death from organ failure is the result. Viruses and neurological diseases are part and parcel of the "cytokine" crisis.

OSA is an immune disorder with autoimmune capabilities. Momma Cass died July 1974 at age 33. She suffered from the obesity of OSA. She died quietly in bed from a heart attack brought about by coronary artery disease. No ham sandwich here. Just crash diets, obesity and OSA.

Reggie White had sarcoid, an autoimmune disease. He died of a fatal heart arrhythmia. He too suffered from OSA and was real big and muscular. I suspect a cytokine storm did the deed in both.

In any event, they died like two ships passing in the night, on the way to a foreign port.

The clues identifying a disease are usually well hidden. If you've heard that scientists are in a way like detectives, it's true. Perhaps not as glamorous as Sherlock Holmes—although a number of scientists have associates (colleagues) or graduate students who could be termed "sidekicks." They seach for the "Holy Grail" of knowledge. Continual sucking the everlasting "Gobstopper", scientists never stop. The past literature is essential to future discoveries. The finding of the ethmoid mast cell was a small step forward for man.

The evidence for neural transmitters is on two levels. The use of neurotoxins (poisons) in the past are used to murder people. One can identify the culprit. Mustard gas, Xylon B, agent orange and dioxin are a few bandits. The neurotrophin growth hormone (NGH) is subtle and practically unknown to most people. This death hormone is produced by ethmoid mast cells. The manufacture of these molecules takes place within the cell. An elaborate assembly-line manufacture takes place. It incorporates particles from the atmosphere signalling the immune genes to rearrange themselves. These genes come from the chromosomes. A little gene here, a little there—and you have immune genes in the future genome. Small glycoproteins function and specialize as chemical mediators. The cytokines run the "show"—the network throughout the body is a cytokine nanonetwork (CNN) This is the origin and cause of sleep apnea.

Mustard gas to destroy nerve tissue was used in World War I. Developed by the German company, Bayer AG, the advanced form was known as HS (Hun Stuff). Mustard gas was also reserved for lesser conflicts where advanced civilized countries know the other side can't relatiate.

An oldie is still a goodie. Advances in cyanide-based insecticides were used by Nazi Germany in the holocast.

The killing fields were extended with the use of agent orange, an exfoliant was introduced during the Korean War. The fields in Korea had luxuriant jungle growth necessitating Agent Orange along the DMZ. The problem was, and is the release of dioxin with the defoliants. Fifty-five gallon orange striped barrels were shipped in Vietnam. Than came the "Rainbow Herbicides". Agents purple, pink, blue and white were shipped. Colour coding made a U.S. Army fashion statement. Agent Orange was outstanding in the Mekong Delta. There was still the problem of dioxin.

The breakdown product of agent orange was deposited in fat and nerve tissue. I was duped here. Nerve deficits of tingling, numbness, pain and weakness of muscles were caused by chemicals.

The body of a nerve cell simulates a "jelly fish." Underwater tenacles are entangled in a gaggle of interlocking connections. The outer myelin sheath and axon are insulated by support cells. These support cells supply nutrients to the myelin and axon. Of course the names Schwann cell and Oligodendrocytes have connotations for PhD. hall of famers! Scientists only. The receptor site in the brain and neuron is the target of the hormone neurotrophin. Thank goodness raising the oxygen level in the body, with a reduction of mast cells does the trick in my patients.

The essential fatty acid or arachidonic acid (AAA) to provide for the signaling of messages in the nerve. My mother gave me a teaspoon of arachidonic acid every morning—she called it cod liver oil. It was foul tasting. In todays world, children call 911 to report their mothers attempt to poison them.

Arachidonic acid is stored in the cell membrane. The mast cell has the enzymes to breakdown AAA into leukotriene 4 (LT4). This lipooxygenase pathway forms cytokines that release the granules of stored biochemical mediators like histamine. LT4 effects are well documented in cellular death of ethmoid cells. Documentation of poisonous effects of chemical was low in the armies and my priorities. Low levels of dioxin in the atmosphere from volcano's, coal fired utilities and metal smelting obscured the clues for increased levels. Particles of dioxin covered the planet and residues contaminated the soil. The Love Canal, as distinguished from the "Love Boat", and the soil about the Allied chemical plants in Baltimore. This legacy of future cancer and neurologic signs and symptoms was missed. The mystery of sleep apnea was camouflaged even as cases of obesity, asthma and diabetes increased exponentially.

In a way, sleep apnea is lurking underneath the common disease we know and love. Immune inflammatory diseases encompass lupus, psoariasis, sarcoid arthritis and chronic fatigue syndrome the neurotransmitters of the mast cell affects the transmission of electrical and chemical signals. From the brain to the smallest nerves the insulation of the nerve sheath sucks up hormones. Neurotrophin is the hormone of sleep apnea. Mast cell in the ethmoid and beyond light up like a Christmas tree. It's kinda—like a pinball machine on a mission. Sleep apneas and related diseases; restless leg syndrome, diabetes, high blood pressure and obesity are kissing cousins.

CHAPTER 16

The River of Shame
Or
The Kepone Dance

The river of shame
Politicians are to blame
Suck in good-old kepone
Your lung turns to stone
Kepone particles up the nose
Sprayed by a garden hose
Kepone affects nerve conduction
With ion and chemical transmission reduction
Misfirings of neural synapses
Kepone can lead to nerve collapse
Kepone takes a health toll
When our body shakes, rattles and rolls

The Appalachian Mountain Rivers connect the waterways in Pennsylvania, Maryland and Virginia. Along the banks of the river are small, medium and large cities with toxic hazardous waste sites. These three states are one giant riverboat system linked by commercial interests. At the confluence of Monongahela and Allegheny rivers, the mighty Ohio River is home to Pittsburgh. Pittsburgh, the number one polluter in the United States, is an old-line industrial giant. The coal powered generators to produce electrical energy spew particulate matter into the sky. The business people with industrial interests in coal-fired power plants have grandfathered any improvements of equipment to clean up the emissions. The owners and CEO's of these coal and steel companies are impressive. They are impeccably dressed. The river cuts through the Appalachian Mountains. There is a sense of brooding gloom from inspecting the waste sites. Documentation of autoimmune disease like OSA, the metabolic syndrome and psoriasis, are frequently observed. My research shows an increase in cases of multiple sclerosis. It's kinda hard to ignore a pandemic of multiple sclerosis. The Cleveland Clinic said better diagnosis was present. Baloney! I've confirmed M.S. patients living on the same block in the local communities. Kepone, the white powder insecticide/pesticide was uncovered from streams in State College (Penn State), PA. There is a large, loosely organized group of autoimmune cases locally. There appears to be a chemical attraction between kepone and the central nervous system. The organochlorinated pesticides have a checkered history.

There is a relationship between the antigenic particles in the atmosphere, the processing of the antigens by lymphocytes and mast cells in the sinus tissues. Cytokine signaling by stimulation of the bone marrow and complex protein production goes forth. The mast cell production facilities for the neuropeptides that affect the nerve cell are stored in the Golgi. There as the rearrangement of genes to provide a blueprint for newer and more complex hormones. The kepone can build up in the fatty tissues, for processing and release of these organic chemicals later.

The slow release of kepone is associated with a chronic nerve condition. Tremors, jerky movements, ringing in the ears, memory loss and muscle weakness are environmental. The half life of kepone is 30 years, and it settles into the sediment in the Bay and its tributaries.

The signaling messages of neuropeptides can affect the nerve plasma membrane. Nerve excitability and neurotransmission is by ion or chemical gradient changes. The nerve fibers (axons) are wrapped in a myelin sheath. A fatty tissue layer of phospholipids control the plasma membrane neurotransmitters. Once the neural transmission has flowing ions the receptor site of the next neuron alters the balance of the ions inside and outside, the synapse continues the process. The flow of nerve continues the process. The flow of nerve excitability is inhibited by kepone. There are neural misfiring; synchronous transmission is screwed up.

If the supporting Schwann cells which provide nutrition to the myelin and axons are totally destroyed, permanent nerve deficits take place. The chemical bonding of kepone is usually a weak one. The structure is reversible. Remove the kepone, and nerve function returns. If the organochemical cause permanent damage, nerve deficits remain. Multiple Sclerosis is an autoimmune disease. My research targets the increasing trends of M.S. in patients exposed to pollutants. I've seen multiple cases on a street to street pattern in Philipsburg, PA.

The James River in Maryland and Virginia know kepone well. The powder was manufactured in Hopewell, VA and initially stored and shipped by Allied Chemical from its distribution center in Race Street, Baltimore. South Baltimore General hospital would experience a surge in cancer cases. Women suffered sterility. Workers suffered tremors, memory loss, slurred speech and other neurologic signs/symptoms.

Kepone was a stable chemical that would contaminate water in the rivers and Chesapeake Bay. Kepone lies in the sediment in the Bay. Fishing was banned and the kepone plant was closed in 1975. Too many workers suffered from "kepone shakes." The taste of contaminated fish is like chicken. It is suspected that fish burgers were served alongside Dinoburgers in Jurassic Park. This tasty morsel was served until the end of the Cretaceous period when the Park permanently shut down.

The Chesapeake Bay was polluted from the effluents releases from kepone plants. How do we know it was kepone? The oyster shells started to vibrate. The edges of the shells were lined parallel. Having the movement of an oscillating serrated electric knife, filleted swimming Bluefish and Rockfish. A massive fish kill ensued. The death of so many fish caught the attention of the Oyster Oversight Committee, a branch of the Federal Government.

The findings of kepone in the Bay initiated a ban on fishing. There were dead and dying flatulent Rockfish. The Environmental Protection Agency was a fact-finding commission with a Mega buck budget. The chemical and fishing industries called on the John Hopkins Public Health Department for background and scientific finding. The first order of business was a brunch at the Hyatt hotel on Baltimore Street

Findings included the monetary consequence of banning kepone, or enforcing a moratorium on fishing is too "political." There was no actual evidence of kepone entering an oyster knocking on the shell. The one note of caution that requires further studies are bubbles rising from the oyster beds to the surface. This was oyster flatulence associated with a fishy stench and fog-like clouds. If you go swimming today and see bubbles, swim like hell; and hold your nose. Their conclusion was kepone causes damage to the oyster nervous system. There was a "dancing oyster" problem identified. First impressions were a relationship between kepones and the nervous system of humans. The organochlorinated pesticides extended into Maryland from small streams in State College, PA. (Penn State)

The use of insecticides may have a moral imperative. Aerial spraying of kepone to kill ants or boll weevils had some value. "Albert's Swarm" of locusts need eradication. Baltimore is infamous for its moral imperative in the wholesale murder of innocent grasshoppers.

The contaminated soil from the Race Street Allied Chemical property was used as landfill. This landfill butted up to the Patapsco River in the Chesapeake. Harbor view is a very valuable property. Kepone and Arsenic forced the City to dedicate a Public Park in 1977. It took paving the landfill, and repeat coverings of topsoil to build a safe bicycle path and basketball courts. The re-sodding of the dump site and topsoil couldn't put Humpty-Dumpty back together again. The scruffy, gnarled shrubs resembled Bonsai trees with brown foliage. Trees appeared to suffer from scurvy. Even the grass looked terminal. The city sold the site to Honeywell. Location, location, location was the new mantra. The John Hopkins Public Health testified kepone was at low levels not to pose a health threat. Arsenic levels also fell to a low. The fix was in. Zoning changes for condo's and townhouses were proposed, docking facilities factored in, and open space recreational areas planned. A hotsy totsy name of Swann Park was proposed. Shopping malls with a Rodeo Drive street sign and address highlighted a showcase of luxurious stores. Condo discounts were offered; no down payment. The New Yuppies took the bait and swallowed.

Unfortunately, the new tenants were developing Neurological diseases. Tremors and involuntary twitching were particular to Swann Park. Two rock songs "Whole lot of Shaking Going On" by Jerry Lee Lewis, and Bill Haley's "Shake Rattle and Roll" were popular. The tenants didn't find them funny. OSA and the metabolic syndrome, asthma, and diabetes were highlights in this first autoimmune park. The water and soil present an ever present danger today.

Kepone can enter our body through the skin or respiratory system. Water that dried out in the soil could develop the cytokines and complex polypeptides to reside in the skin, and nervous tissue. The sediment from the bay would dry up, and the kepone fibers breached the atmosphere. Again autoimmune systemic diseases would multiply. Stores of kepone in fat tissue would be released slowly.

The Susquehanna River, at Three Mile Island near Harrisburg, PA., had a nuclear accident. Radiation was leaked and iodine-131 was carried into the Chesapeake. The highest radon concentrations lead to increased cancer rates. 1979 was a bad year for lung cancer along the Appalachian Rivers. Kepone was to join the pollutants in the Chesapeake Bay. The sudden appearance of the five eyed opalina with a vacuum mouth to suck up radioactive debris from the Bay floor was a taxon. The trilobite from the Devonian period only had a brief appearance. The radiation caused the trilobites to light up. The shiny eyeballs attracted other predators.

Unfortunately, the Maryland Blue Crab population was decimated. The soft shell crabs (peelers) never developed hard shells. Without a hard outer shell, they developed "crab burns"; kinda like a sunburn. The blue color turned red and they turned onto their backs with crab legs sticking straight upwards. The crab legs could easily be removed from their sockets. This was not a sign of crab rot, but of a crab cooked in pollutants. Croaking crabs and trilobites running amok; who could ask for anything more.

Zyklon-B was developed as a pesticide by Fritz Habor, a German Jew. Developed as a pesticide for delousing clothing and preventing typhus, it was sold to the chemical giant I. G. Farben in 1930. Haber emigrated and the Jews were gassed.

In the United States, Zyklon-B was used for delousing Mexican farm hands clothing and washing down freight cars. The naked bodies were sprayed with the toxic fumigants like DDT. Zyklon-B is absorbed through the skin sinuses and lungs. The drenching of clothing with Zyklon-B onto a wet naked body from fumigants is quite cruel. Acute toxicity and death from Zyklon-B would be unacceptable. Possible death, birth defects, cancer and autoimmune disease would haunt the immigration authorities and Mexican-American relations. The American government built a first-class disinfection plant in 1938. The Nazi's admired the plants design. It was to be modified from a showcase of exterminating lice to more sinister use. Zyklon-B was used to murder millions in the death camps.

American chemists are clever. They were able to synthesize an insecticide and fungicide that is long lasting and very stable. Kepone is a wonder drug. It was introduced in 1966 for use in ant baits and banned in 1975. Kepone persists in the environment today. It's not much of a success story.

The United States has multiple world class toxic dump sites. Others include Ranipot, India; home to a factory that produces tanning chemicals and dumps tons of waste into vacant, unsecured areas. Another member of the top ten polluters is the Kabwe Lead Mine in Zambia. Sickness around toxic sites start with the children. China is on a roll. As the pollutants increase in the big cities, a cloud envelopes Planet Earth. It isn't the morning dew. The diseases increase, and the political games continue. Ask me "for whom does the bell toll; it tolls for the children!'

Errigh La Boo
1740 Wentworth Ave
Balto. Md 21234
410 258-4946

CHAPTER 17

Errigh La Boo, the CPAP—Man

Meet Errigh La Boo, bravest of them all
CPAP—Man heard Doctor Newberg's call
An RDI of 103 is "off the wall"
No memory to think or crawl
Standard treatments over a long time
Perpetuates the sleep apnea crime
Curse this machine, I want the cure
Put CPAP into the drawer
Errichs surgery was quasi—taboo
All's well with Errigh La Boo

Errigh La Boo was first seen in the Baltimore office 5/2/96 for severe OSA. In spite of CPAP for 6 years, he was nodding off with worsening XDS. His weight increased to 243 pounds. A fishing buddy from a trip referred Errigh. Consultation with other post operative patients of mine convinced Errigh to proceed with my new surgery. A pattern of curing sleep apnea was emergings.

Physical examination showed the usual flabby and flaccid throat tissues. The uvula and soft palate were accompanied by rather small (2+) tonsils hanging down like worn-out socks. He had a large tongue and epiglottis. A sleep study from John Hopkins in 1990 showed an RDI of 103 with a mean oxygen level of 92%. Oxyen fell to 72% and there was no stage 3 or 4 restorative sleep. His condition was deteriorating health-wise. The metabolic syndrome was worsening.

He had a long history of allergies. Skin testing showed a potpourri of positive skin reactions. This would require serum and desensitization. The usual gaggle of allergy medicines included anti-histamines, decongestants; seldane was frequent. Beconase, a cortisone nasal spray was frequent.

Errigh hated the CPAP. It was uncomfortable and caused eye irritations including dry eye. A sore nose. The resemblance to a "Borg" device scared the children at first. Errigh might have been on the Planet Mongo when guests came over. They didn't want to stay overnight.

The surgery—the Full Monty—was 6/7/96 for the throat surgery, and completed with bilateral ethmoidectomy 6/14/96.

The surgery was quite successful. The snoring and sleep-disordered-breathing were immediately gone. The children weren't totally happy because the CPAP sound rocked them to sleep And Errigh sang "Good-by CPAP, see you in my dreams".

Errigh and the Missus discuss the surgery–interviewed September 22, 2007

I discussed the tracheostomy with my wife but it was scary not breathing without a track. And if I had to do it all over again; yes—in a heartbeat. My voice was pretty low, but soon the tongue heals and the quality comes back.

The first two or three days were the most uncomfortable, mostly from the throat surgery. After that there was steady progression. I have to eat a bit slower and if I drink incorrectly, the fluid comes out my nose.

The question is how is your snoring now and after the operation? What kind of difference has the operation made? I do not snore or use the CPAP machine. Dr. Newberg is going to verify this through a sleep study.

Mrs. La Boo noted the episodes of stopping breathing; a total of 20 minutes out of each hour. We had an HMO and they didn't want to give us the machine after the sleep study in 1990. The cause was the expense. I got on the phone and he had it in two weeks.

Besides the snoring and sleep apnea he was tired all the time. I used to joke and exaggerate that when he was snoring the room would be sucking in and out. I told him he was better off declaring his love before finding out he snored. I would think twice before marrying him. He's not snoring at all. Its unbelievable, because I don't hear a sound. A few times, I've gone to the room at 2:00 or 3:00 in the morning and sat down real close and realized there was no sound coming from him.

Erigh has severe allergies. The medicines didn't work after time. He had nasal blockages. He was allergic to everything. We have a cat but we'll keep the cat and get rid of you.

Erigh and his wife were interviewed September 22, 2007 at a steak house in Baltimore. The results from the surgery are wonderful. No snoring, sleep apnea or tiredness. Weight is about the same. Further social history shows Errigh was active military during Vietnams

Army Corp. of Engineers on assignment to Cameron Bay in 1971.

There is no snoring or sleep apnea. There are no regrets. Allergy shots continue.

There are 4 children, the oldest is 40 who snores and has allergies. One of the two daughters, age 24 is overweight with high blood pressure. She has two young children, one with allergies and asthma. A young teenage son finishing high school is normal.

One can see a definite correlation been allergies and sleep apnea. The seven patients, the magnificent seven, have their skin testing and allergies chronicled.

The sleep studies post-operative were basically normal. A full sleep study one month from surgery, on 7/11/96 showed and RDi of 6 and oxygen baseline of 95%. Three years later, 6/22/99 a full sleep study by an attended in—laboratory sleep center showed an RDI of 2.5 a baseline of O_2 98% with a low O_2 of 96%. Sleep architecture was restored with stages 1, 2, 3, 4 and REM. His clinical findings mirror the sleep studies. Errigh and I both got lucky.

Yes, Errich had filet mignon and his wife sea bass. They rejected a spinach salad. Errigh scarfed down the fillet quickly.

Post-operative history shows

Errich was doing real well until 2004 when he fainted and fell at work. An arrhythmia and slow heart beat required a pace maker defibrillator. Post-operatively, he had a pneumothorax treated by chest tube. In 2006, heart disease and weight gain caused congestive heart failure. He is on Lasix and Toprol. Errigh is a maven of reasoned thought when OSA is complicated by the metabolic syndrome, he is an advisor to the public. He leaves his phone number and address to answer questions. He feels strongly about his treatment and pledges to help others. Two close friends of Errigh recently had unsuccessful sleep apnea surgery in Baltimore by other physicians. (You can lead a horse to water but . . . .)

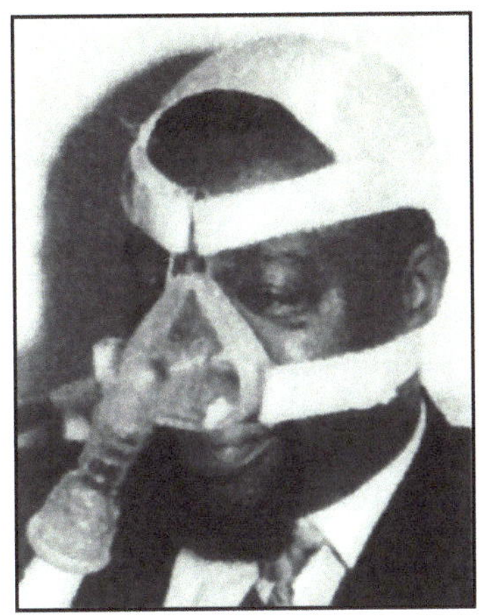

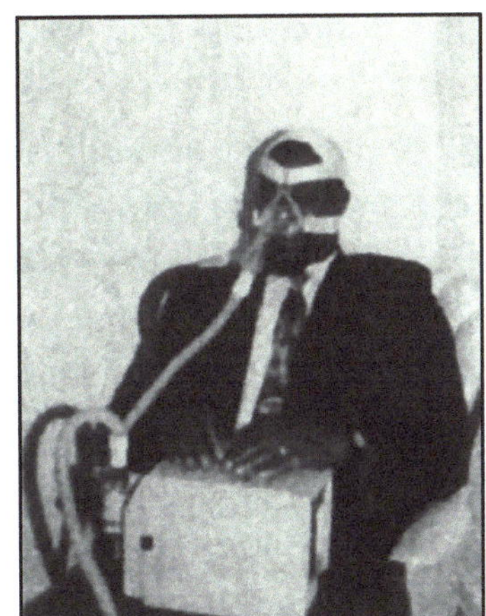

from Snore and Roar, 1996
Errigh La Boo
CPAP – Man

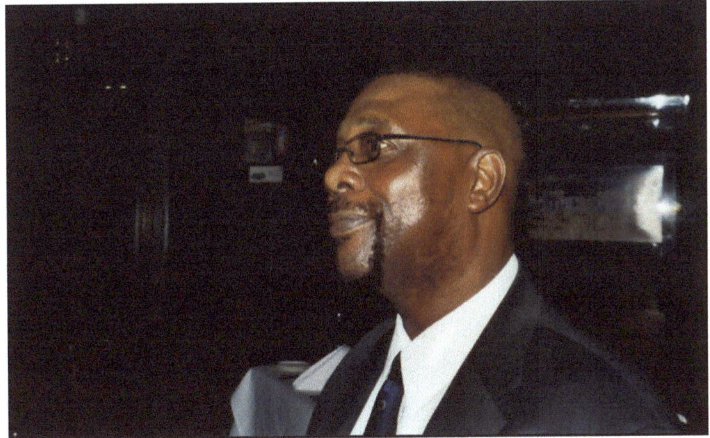

Errigh La Boo
Sept 22, 2007

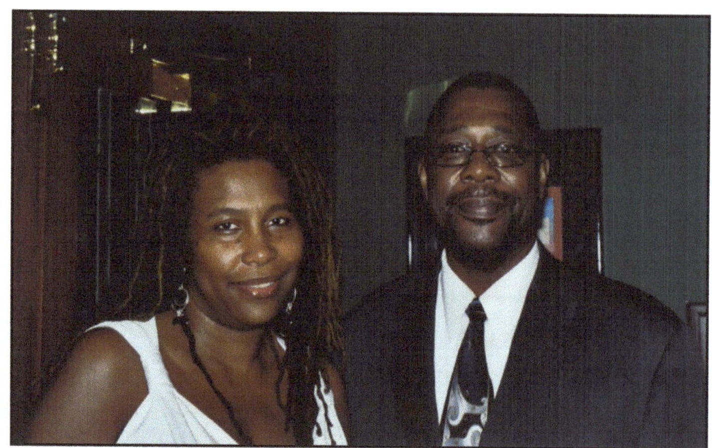

Errigh la Boo and wife
Sept 22, 2007

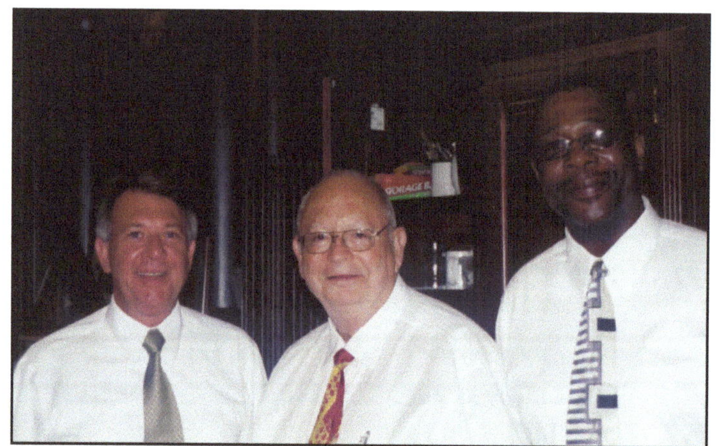

right to left: Errigh La Boo, Dr. Lewis Newberg, John Wozniak - State Senator and "Full Monty" graduate

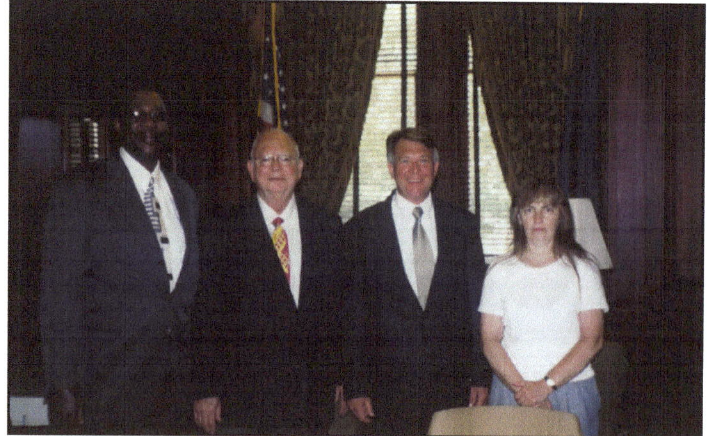

State Senator John Wozniak, a full Monty graduate, Dr. Lewis Newberg, Errigh La Boo, Karen Blair, Administrator, Philipsburg Hospital

CHAPTER 18

Serendipity

Severe sleep-disordered breathing makes one cry
Addition of the metabolic syndrome prepares them to die
My hypothesis and theory tell
The sleep apnea hormone is produce in the mast cell
Neurotrophic Growth Hormone is supported by reversible ligands
Neural bonds with the strength of a rubber band
Mirror, mirror on the wall
Who can cure them all?
I made the call
Now all shop at the mall

I suffer from OSA. Many of the accoutrements of the metabolic syndrome have ravaged my body. OSA's sleep-disordered-breathing and excessive daytime sleepiness started the metabolic process. High blood pressure was a sentinel sign in progression of the disease. This is an ominous finding; my surgery will cure most stages. Remove ethmoid cells, raise blood oxygen levels and Nirvana. The treatment with CPAP doesn't reverse high blood pressure. High blood pressure medicine is just a band aid in the treatment. Obesity, coronary artery disease with dyslipidemia and congestive heart failure are consequences in OSA. Other autoimmune conditions like psoriasis and insulin resistant diabetes show the wide range of immune responses. The recent finding of Leptin, the fat hormone, provides some hope in future research projects. The fat hormone is produced by the adipocyte (fat cell) in the bone marrow, and expands the fat stores in the belly. There are high blood levels of Leptin in OSA patients but manipulation of fat stores hasn't cured OSA. My levels are probably on the ceiling. The increase of Leptin plasma levels should lead to a decrease in fat stores. But the satiety gene is competing at the brains receptor sites with other neuropeptides. All these hormones were forming pathological base for OSA. The addition of my total ethmoid operation was yielding good long-term cure rates. Did I measure the Leptin levels in my patients? No! There was a severe lack of resources. University centers keeping their technology under strict control; no Leptin could be measured. But my why? and how? of OSA was proceeding quite well. I was getting worse.

My sleep apnea condition deteriorated and two heart attacks led to coronary bypass surgery. In 1996, I awoke from a sound sleep with a message and information. I lived in a townhouse in Chaddsford, PA. It was 2 AM and I stumbled to the top of the stairs with the grey carpeting. My bedroom was on the second floor. The telepathic message said . . . "Write it, and it will come." Write what? What will come? Was it watching too many DVD's including Field of Dreams. I sensed the cure for OSA was related to the ethmoid operation. The combination of ethmoid surgery combined with a modified UPPP (throat) surgery at the same hospitalization was the way to go. These messages were to initiate the greatest stories I ever told. The bandages on my chest still covered the gaping wounds of open heart surgery at Washington Hospital Center.

Maybe residual anesthesia; perhaps the whole episode was a dream. I walked slowly down the steps into the kitchen. Write a book. Poppycock!

It took two years to write the book "Snore or Roar." I can't type, probably can't write either; wrote it by hand, word by word. It was an enjoyable read and quite informational. Being a surgeon, not a bookseller, most copies were given away free to my patients. Unconsciously, the book goosed an incentive from my curiosity. I sent part of three surgical ethmoid specimens from OSA patients to the University of Maryland for light and electron microscopy.

Serendipity. Dr. Ling, Pathologist at Harbor Hospital called me back in 1996 to tell me the ethmoid tissue in the three OSA patients were flooded with mast cells. These three cases gave reasoned thought to the concept of an immune response in OSA patients. Experimental data of the third kind is irrefutable. The mast cell is OSA.

The refinement of the procedure into a one hospital admission called the "Full Monty." All patients with moderate to severe OSA started with Errigh LaBoo in 1996 were operated this way. The Full Monty became my standard throat operation with the accompanying bilateral ethmoid operation. Now you know the rest of the story.

The production of hormones from amino acids into complex neuropeptides including pheromones and neutrophin is old hat. Pheromones, the sex hormones, have graduated from a reproductive smell to a perfume bottle. The assembly line production in the mast cell by the endoplasmic reticulum, Golgi apparatus and ribosome was copied by the "Garment District" in New York. Under the duel influences of genetic traits, and the environmental factor of gene rearrangement, a dynamic ever-changing process in the genome was underway.

I suspect a new sushi superantigen. A reconfigured antigen was environmental. Perhaps protein fragments with sesame seeds or fish roe inside out, was environmental. The ensuing nasal inflammation sent new signals through the cytokine nanonetwork (CNN). The processing by the B and T cells and the newly discovered Leptin hormone became cytokine driven. This was a microcosm of the old prehistoric Devonian period where genes ran amok. This new neurotrophin growth hormone was conceived by DNA and RNA gene rearrangement from environmental clues. This hormone would diffuse pass the blood brain barrier to a receptor site in a brain or neuron cell. There might be emailing between the ethmoid mast cells, and mast cells of the nerve cell. These endogenous mast cells may contribute to misfiring of neural impulses. The receptor sites compete for natural hormones. The abnormal NTG, in the presence of a lowered oxygen level will lead to, and contribute to progressive abnormalities in nerve conduction. Hence, sleep-disordered-breathing is a self fulfilling prophesy. The progression of malfunctioning neural circuits may be associated with restless leg syndrome. All the soft epithelial cells were killed and replaced by bone. Here was sclerosis.

Addition of the Magnificent Seven (the seven samurai warriors) volunteered to share their experiences. They feel an obligation. All were CPAP wearers with severe OSA and the metabolic syndrome. The signs/symptoms of a cure could be observed and measured by long-term follow-up sleep studies. My innovative surgery worked quite well.

There is so much hanky-panky in results today. Outright fraud is hard to recognize. My patients want to help patients with OSA and have volunteered their privacy. They will accept phone calls. All seven patients were cherry-picked for severity of their disease and CPAP users. It's easy to observe a good result. They are happy to share personal data. Their clinical improvement of signs and symptoms of OSA are impressive. The CPAP machines have been long gone.

James Friday's (case #1) wife Agnes worked in the Philipsburg office. Her daughter Dawn then took over as secretary. Kim Yaple, secretary, keeps track of all pre and post-operative patients. Is she honest? She's from the Moshannon Valley in PA. That says it all!

The Magnificent Seven know OSA is the mast cell. Though dating from prehistoric times, the neurotrophs hormone is produced in Nasty Masty. The molecular modeling of complex proteins including neuropeptides, is from the immune system. Patients have benefited from this knowledge. They enjoy the enlarged photo of a mast cell in OSA that sits on my desk.

CHAPTER 19

The Three Amigo's

The Three Amigo's
Are genuine heroes
Three special patients with severe OSA
Underwent surgery in the good old USA
The surgeon didn't have a clue
Light and Electron Microscopy of ethmoid tissue
Mast cells from the immune system were believed
The cure of OSA could be achieved
The three patients knew the reason why
It was their choice to do or die
Was the new operation nonsense
To risk loss of my medical license
How do you like your eggs in the morning?
I like mine with a kiss!

From the B-cell came a four protein immunoglobulin molecule. Gene rearrangement in the immune system produces antibodies. Immunoglobulin antibody has 2 heavy chains and 2 light chains. Lymphocytes are the only cells in the body that rearranges genes from sushi rolls. Sushi genes come from the variety of rolls in the menu. The immunoglobulin of the B lymphocyte switches from IgG to IgE antibody. Blood plasma cells protection also produce IgE. Two sources of supply are good.

The IgE antibody drops anchor into the surface of an ethmoid tissue mast cell. I uncovered the hidden world of mast cells flooding and poisoning ethmoid tissues. This discovery would produce the roadmap to cure OSA.

Sleep-disordered-breathing disappeared following my patients surgeries. The release of this hormone from falling production in the ethmoid cells with increasing oxygen levels is the theory of OSA. OSA is reversible. I wonder if the destruction of neuron and Schwann cells is reversible/ preventable in multiple sclerosis.

The role of the mast cell in OSA never crossed my mind before the three patients were operated at South Chester County Medical Center. My surgery of combining ethmoidectomy with throat surgery was unique. The "how and why" of OSA would be answered by curing patients. The three amigos made history. They were also cured. This was fun.

Table 1 shows the three patients with OSA operated in 1996. Because of my curiousity, the ethmoid tissue was divided in half at Southern Chester Medical Society and transported by me to the University of Maryland for light and electron microscopy. The pathologist at Harbor hospital contacted a fellow pathologist for a favor. As part of his routine pathologies, he ran my tissues that were preserved in icebox containers from Walmart. The specimens were placed in pathology containers at the university.

Doctor Ling called me to announce mast cells infiltrating and flooding the ethmoid tissues in all three patients. My first thought was "what are mast cells?" Why are they here? How did they get here? Do they relate to OSA?

The refinement of the procedure into a one hospital admission is called the "Full Monty." All patients with moderate to severe OSA started with Errigh La Boo in 1996 were operated this way. The Full Monty became my standard throat operation with the accompanying bilateral ethmoid operation. Now you know the rest of the story.

The three amigo's operated in 1996 had light and electron microscopy of their ethmoid tissue. Why did I send tissue to the University? No idea—perhaps curiousity. Perhaps it was time for sleep apnea to show it's secret to the world.

Mast cell 101 started in 1996. Everything you always wanted to know but were too afraid (or asleep) to ask your biology teacher. Half the ethmoid tissue in the three cases operated at Southern Chester County Medical Center were placed in separate containers. They were placed in dry ice and transported by me to the University of Maryland. The tissue removed by me at the time of surgery was from the bulla ethmoidalis, and extending through the ground lamella into the posterior ethmoid.

The readings of ethmoid tissue for mast cells were performed by Board-certified pathologists at the University of Maryland. Doctor Virginia Ling at Harbor hospital confirmed the readings and called me. Not quite as exciting a read as the latest Harry Potter book, but still an interesting read. Well. To the pathologists at least.

Specimens to be examined by light microscopy were received in the histology laboratory and assigned surgical pathology numbers. Each specimen was gently squeezed (I promise gently! We don't need a lawsuit on behalf of the specimens here) with forceps while being drawn across four slides. Staining with hematoxylin and eosin. This whole process you find riveting, I'm sure.

A Giemesa stain was ordered to highlight the mast cell granules. Different chemicals allowed the Giemsa stain to these slides, microphotographs were taken by neoflar lens (16/0.40) under high-power magnification (40x). (Think of it as a recipe. Scientists could have their own cooking shows—shouting a BAM! with each new ingredient . . . . although, please don't try and make it at home. And here we go.)

Light Microscopy

<u>Normal Tissue</u>: (Also known as the people who are probaly not reading this book)

Light microscopy of normal ethmoid tissue shows a ciliated pseudostratified columnar epithelium (dark cell), with goblet (mucus) cells. They are clear and foamy. The ratio of ciliated cells to goblet cells are 1:1. There are variations. A big variation suggests the possibility some of the goblet cells got distracted and wandered off from specimen to specimen. The layer of cells is supported by a light pink basement membrane. (A light pink basement . . . . doesn't sound like somewhere you would want to be on a Friday night)

<u>Patient Tissue</u>: Or the people with no friends once the sun sets

Light microscopy of the ethmoid sinus mucosa in all three OSA patients showed changes consistent with acute or chronic inflammation. The lining of the epithelium in each case showed ciliated columnar cells and decreased goblet cells (<u>Figs. 1, 2</u>) numerous mast cells were found in all specimens. (You get all that? Basically, I'm trying to tell you the patient cells were different.

Acute inflammatory cells in lamina propria (under the pink basement membrane) are mast cells. A lonely mucus cell with bubbles is front row center. There are none to few mucus cells per highpowered field (hpf). The lamina propria consists of fibrosis and collagen deposition (a filler). The mast cells have reddish cytoplasm with a nice purple nucleus—a big fat one is in the center. (I guess the more appropriate term would be, "A big boned one is in the center." We really need to be careful around those "Cell Rights" people. Where have all the goblet cells gone (0 per hpf)? Why are mast cells here? These are questions that will continue to haunt you from night to night, I'm sure. Better read on.

Figure 3 shows a decrease in the seromucinous component of glands in the lamina propria. Giema staining showed that the cytoplasm was packed with basophilic granules that are known to contain preformed histamine. Granules with preformed mediators are triggered by activation of the mast cell to release granules that are local poisons; vasoactive amines (histamine) and proteases. Tissue injury to the cell, or surrounding cells may lead to death of the cell. (See? See what I did? I'm trying to use a mystery for you to keep reading. Is it working?)

Figure 4

Light microscopy shows dystrophic calcification in the lamina propria of OSA patient's ethmoid tissue. Acute inflammation by mast cells complicated by the breakdown of arachidonic acid into a cascade of products. Cytokines, local chemical messengers signal the cascade. The leukotrienes (LT4) has the ability to kill tissues—and to release mucus. Death of goblet (mucus) cells leaves a skeleton which is filled in by calcium salts and other minerals. Calcification of the tissues makes curretting them at surgery more difficult. The death of tissue leads to a shrinking volume to the ethmoid sinus. The normal aeration is disturbed and nasal function is reduced. Chronic mouth breathing, and nasal obstruction are long-term effects compatible with OSA. The sclerosis seen on a lateral planigram in chronic mastoid disease is similar to the ethmoid. The similar phenomenom of sclerosis cannot be seen well on routine sinus or CT of the ethmoids because of overlapping soft tissues and bone. It will depend on a future CT—three dimensional ethmoid technique. (What can I say? The CT—three dimensional ethmoid technique is a show off.)

Electron Microscopy Examination

The tissues were prepared in the usual way for electron scanning. Semi thin sections were staired with toluidine blue and examined under the light microscope to select areas for thin sectioning. Thin sections (60 nm—80 nm) were staired with uranyl acetate—lead citrate and examined with a JOEL 100B transmission electron microscope at 60 KeV. The ethmoid tissue samples of three OSA patients were studied and compared to normal ethmoid tissue. (Once again . . . . I've included a step-by-step process, but please don't try this at home. On another note, do any readers think there would be a profit in a science experiment modeled like a cooking show? Yes? No? Things to think about as we continue to the analysis . . . .)

Normal Tissue: or the people most of the readers are jealous of

Under electron microscopy, the normal ethmoid epithelium was composed of three different types of cells: basal, ciliated, and goblet Ratio of goblet cells to ciliated cells is 1:1. Normal ciliated pseudostratified columnar cells are squeezed between large goblet cells. (Figure 5).

The goblet cells, located in the middle and apical layers of the epithelium, contain large and electron-lucent mucus granules with faint reticulated contents. They are the large bull's eye-shaped structures. (I hope some readers didn't get too excited at the bull's-eye comparison hoping we might stray off and start talking about bulls . . . . that was just to tease you. We're continuing with science lingo now).

The goblet cells squeeze the ciliated cells (basically . . . . these two were not friends. Or at least the goblet cells had stronger feelings toward the ciliated cells. You know how it goes). The lamina propria contains loosely arranged fibroblasts, thin walled vessels, seromucinous glands, lymphocytes, eosinophils, and mast cells (Still with me after that list? I'm impressed).

Patient Tissue: Or those who were forced to room alone in college

Electron microscopy shows a marked atrophy and decrease in the number of goblet cells in the ethmoid tissue of all three patients, thus examined (Figure 6). The ratio of goblet to ciliated cells are 1:2 The goblet cells had fewer mucus granules than normal tissue. (Mucus granules . . . . so who is going to eat dinner soon after reading this?) Ciliated cells are no longer being squeezed, opposite of what was seen in normal tissue. (Now, its the ciliated cells with stronger feelings for the goblet cells). These findings are classical effects of the leukotrienes on mucus cells.

Figure 7

Electron microscopy showing a mast cell with scroll rich granules. They resemble a bundle of torahs. The centers of the granules contain dense particles. Other, lighter colored granules have a regular crystalline pattern

The mast cell was confused by the blood basophil. Supposedly, a blood basophil was to become a tissue mast cell. We know this is incorrect. The blood basophil has a polylobed (multi headed) nucleus—resembling 2 or 3 egg yolks joined in one egg. (Once again, don't get too excited by the references to more exciting things. We still have science to chat about. On another note, how sad is it that eggs are considered the most interesting point of this paragraph?).

Figure 8

Electron microscopy of patients mast cell showing grating / lattice structure (rough endoplasmic reticulum cisterna) in granules. Nuclear membrane at bottom of photo has dense particles; some structures resemble owls eyes;

See what I'm doing now. First a mystery, now an enthusiastic cheer. (All saying . . . . read on please)

Fig 1

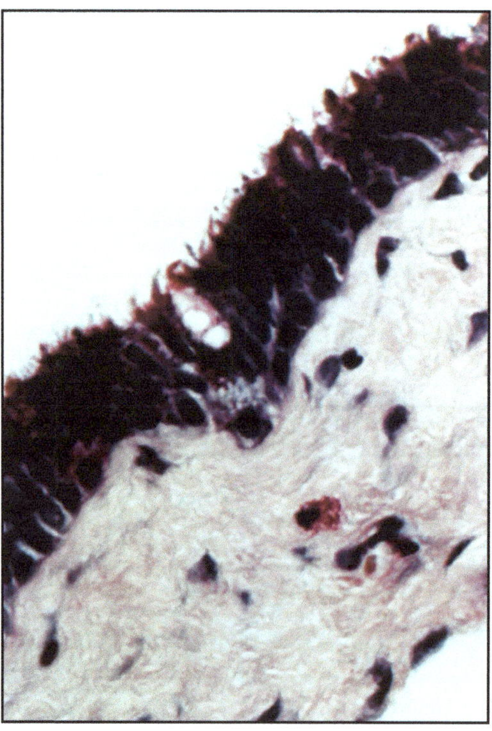

OSA patient's ethmoid tissue under light microscopy, using neofluar lens 16/0.40 under 40X maginification per HPF. Hematoxylin-eosin (H&E) staining of cytoplasm; Giernsa staining for mast cells. Epithelium shows a decrease in goblet cell are less vacuolated. Ciliated cells are more cuboidal and eosinophilic; cilia are shorter, haphazardly oriented. Acute inflammatory cell in lamina propria is mast cell.

Fig 2

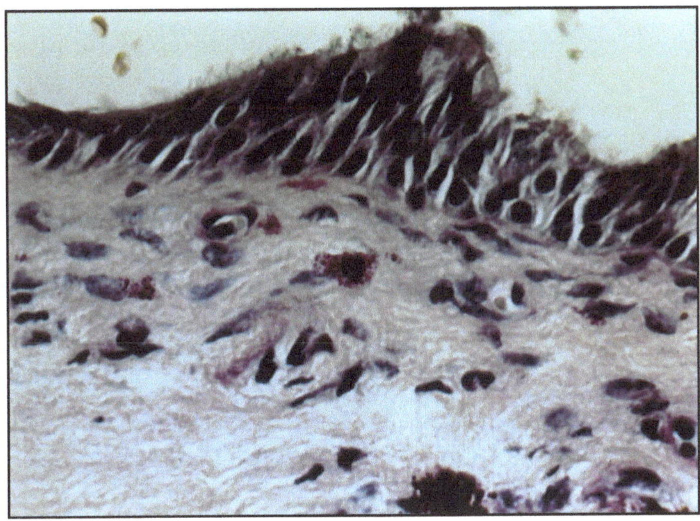

Light microscopy of OSA patient's ethmoid tissue shows absence of goblet cells; increased mast cells in submucosa and lamina propria; Giemsa stain shows cytoplasm of mast cells packed with basophilic granules.

Fig 3

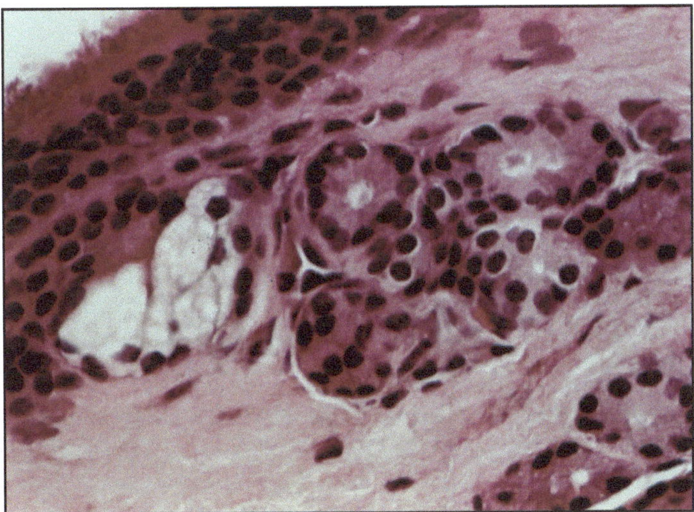

Light microscopy of OSA patient's ethmoid tissue shows a decrease in the seromucinous component of glands in lamina propria.

Fig 4

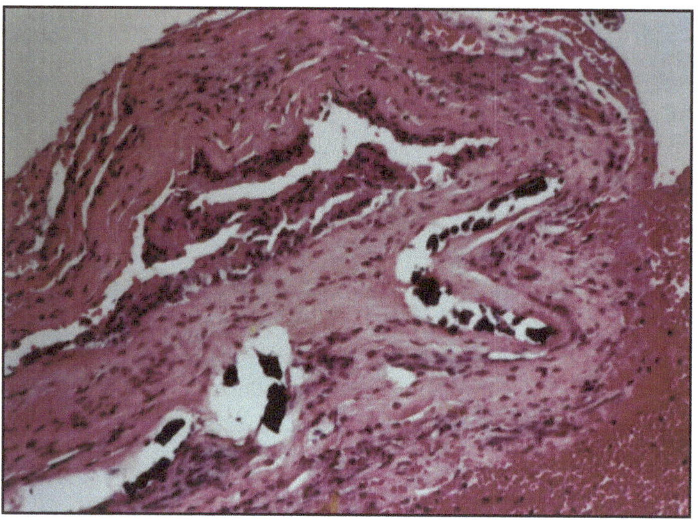

A focus of dystrophic calcification in the lamina propria of patients ethmoid tissue; seen when dead cells and cellular debris are not promptly destroyed and reabsorbed. They attract calcium salts and other minerals that become calcified. Clinically manifested as sclerosis and a decreased volume of ethmoid tissue found at ethmoidectomy in OSA patients.

Fig 5

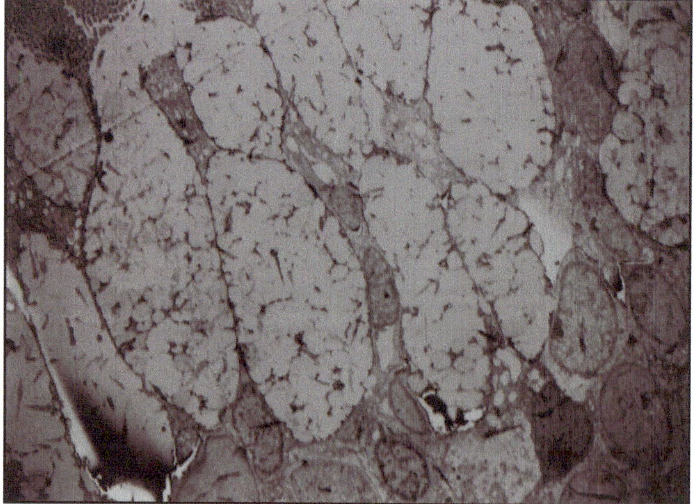

Electron micrsocopy of ethmoid tissue from normal control show three types of cells, basal, ciliated cells is 1:1. Normal ciliated pseudostratified cells are squeezed between large goblet cells.

Fig 6

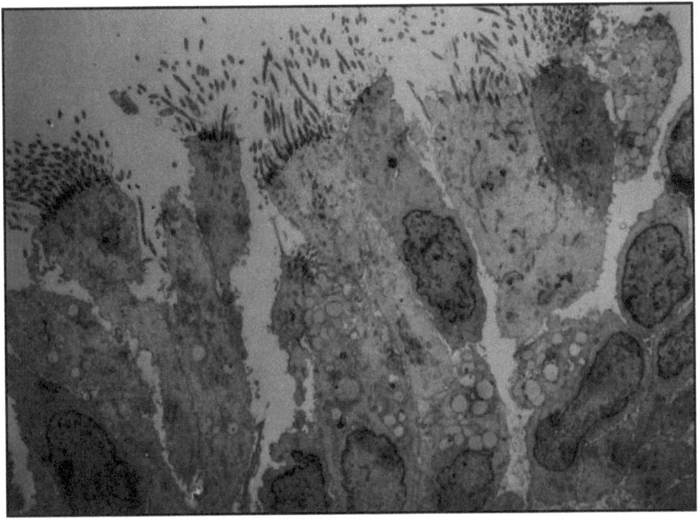

Electron microscopy of OSA patients shows atrophy and decreased number of goblet cells. Ratio of goblet to ciliated pseudostratified columnar cells is now 1:2 or 3:10, compared to normal ratio if 1:1. Nucleus of affected goblet cell is not squeezed and appears alone. Few mucous granules are seen in goblet cells.

Fig 7

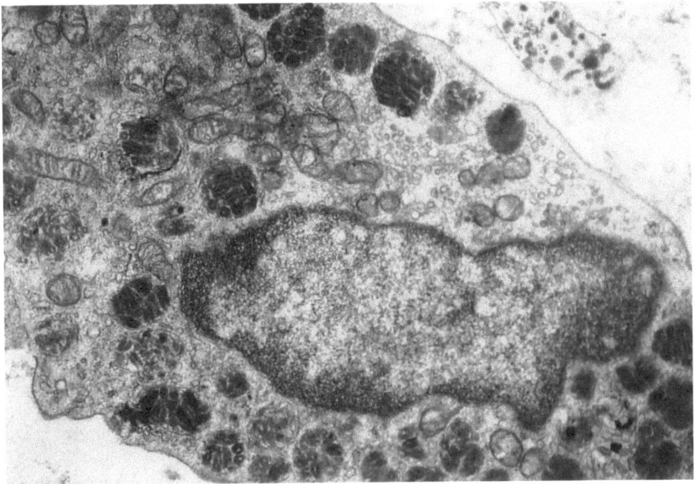

Electron microscopy showing a mast cell with scroll rich granules. They resemble a bundle of torahs. The nucleus is prominent.

Fig 8

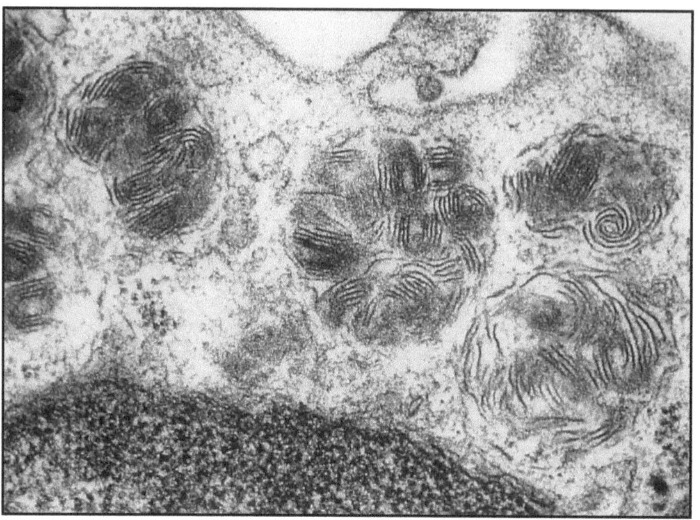

Electron microscopy of a patient mast cell showing grating/lattice in granules; what appears to be "owls" eyes on right. Cisterna of rough endoplasmic reticulum and endoplasmic prominent, nuclear membrane and nucleus with dense particles at bottom.

Table 1. Three patients with OSA in Early 1996 — Light and Electron Microscopy of Ethmoid Tissue

Patient	Environmental History	Age	Respiratory Distress Index (RDI)
A	Atopic; previous job exposure to organic chemicals; ex-smoker; hypertensive; coronary a. disease with pacemaker; CPAP for years	56	61
B	No atopy	50	36
C	No atopy; hx of asthma; non-smoker	37	20.5

CHAPTER 20

The Full Monty – Part I

Newberg's Modified UPPP Operation

Abnormal throat anatomy in snoring and sleep apnea
Aren't the design of Utopia
Floppy uvula and soft palate falls downwards
During sleep the large tongue drops backwards
It's a cut here, a slash there
Then the laser everywhere
This sounds like butchery
Just a refinement of modern surgery

Fig 9

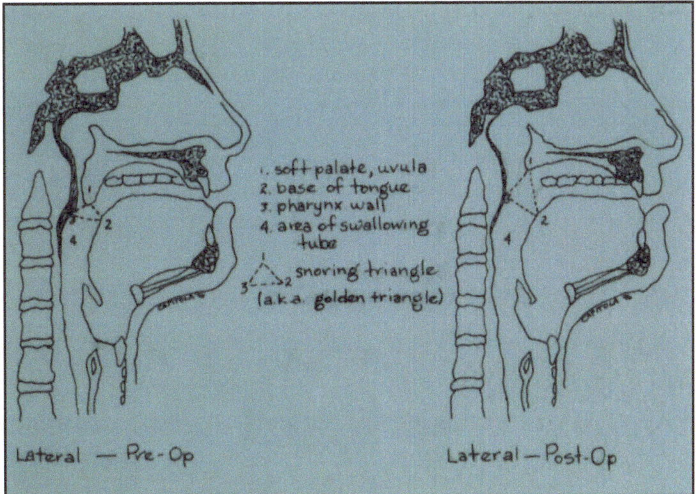

-taken from 1996 Snore or Roar
Pre and post OP UPPP
1-3 enlargement of snoring aka golden triangle
5 Reduction of epiglottis

Evaluation and surgical treatment of habitual snoring stated in 1963, in Noda City, Japan. Noda City is a suburb of Tokyo, and the home of the manufacture of Kikkoman soy sauce. Sake is also made there. These sauces and booze were better known than the partial uvulectomy operation pioneered by Doctor T Ikematsu. 1500 patients, mostly female, underwent this local outpatient surgical procedure from 1963-83. The results in habitual snoring were never documented. Observations on numbers and percentages, short and long-term improvement, and temporary or permanent cures were unknown.

Another 150 patients from the 1963-7 period did have an attempt at statistics for improvement in snoring. Incredibly 81%, 4 out of 5 patients who had the procedure on the uvula and/or soft palate showed success. Are these phantom numbers for snoring alone? Jabberwocky is thy name. It surfaces that fully 60% of Ikematsu's 150 patients were lost to follow up.

The floppy, thinned out, and non-functioning throat tissues were mimsy twins. The uvula and soft palate vibrate in the wind. These anatomical flopperoo's contributed to an accompanying negative upper airway pressure. The pressures developed from the tip of the nose downward into the depths of the throat. A hypothesis, which is just an educated "guess", reinforced the dogma throat tissues cause OSA.

What went wrong? My patients act upon the moral authority implied in a physician's knowledge. The disease vector of a mosquito, or bacteria or virus is understandable when viewed in the context of a specific disease. And if there is no vector, physicians have to take an educated guess. The patient is not a dork, geek or retard. He places his blind trust in physicians as experts in sleep apnea. The lack of an origin or cause of OSA places physician and patient at risk. If the surgery is perceived as ineffective, or unnecessary, the trust will fall. The bond between physician and patient in moderate to severe OSA surgical treatment is broken. A cure rate that approaches zero should not be done. Indeed, most cases of severe OSA are referred for CPAP machines. And the long-term cure rate for the standard UPPP operation in moderate to severe OSA does approach zero.

The surgical results in snoring were temporary. The slicing, freezing, burning, lasering or dicing of the uvula, soft palate didn't do the job. Then came strengthening the throat tissues with implants and other foreign materials. It was hope that I underwent 2 Laser-Assisted Uvulopalatoplasties (LAUP). Snoring was relieved short-term and OSA was unchanged. Multiple visits and procedures were the answer. The algorithm became the chosen or preferred procedure leading to multiple procedures. Documentation of the multiple operations on a flow sheet started with the locally invasive uvula/soft palate surgery. The results would start "at the top" and "go down" to the bottom.

This sounded like a con, a hip hop formula to cure OSA. The algorithm gave a well-defined instructions to complete the task to cure OSA. There was almost incorporation of randomness into the desperation of an algorithm. It sounded that failure was assured. Since there's no cure here, or there, let's operate everywhere. This is a formula for disaster. As my father put things into perspective, "It's the old, who shot Willie approach!" Since the scientific basis was only an educated guess, an unproven hypothesis, it represented the rope-a-dope maneuver. Where were the Medical Society authorities? Medical politicians, hospital administrators and lawyers were willing hostages to this explosion of additional surgeries. Medical Society double-speak justified the algorithm. If at first you don't succeed, try and try again.

If physicians are perceived as performing unnecessary or unproven medical procedures for monetary gain, then their moral authority is lost. An attitude of "who are you to question us," we're the experts and have all the answers, is a superior condescending attitude. The physician whose quest is for money, and yet desires the prestige, will soon have neither. Medicine is far too important, and too expensive to allow untried, useless procedures. Basic research and observable facts were bypassed. A religious chant for OSA surgery rooted in witchcraft doesn't cut it.

The surgery developed by Ikematsu for habitual snoring would be upgraded to the much more extensive uvulopalatopharyngoplasty (UPPP) operation. (Figure 9) Developed by Doctor S. Fujita at the Henry Ford Hospital in Detroit, it involved extensive tissue removal with reconstruction of throat tissues. Unfortunately, an algorithm once started, never met a surgeon it didn't like. Surgery from the uvula, soft palate would be extended to the surrounding tonsils, tonsillar pillars and other redundant tissue.

These were considered fair game. Poor results with the standard UPPP led me to modify the basic operation to include the base of the tongue. Figure 9 shows the snoring triangle after surgery. This is nicknamed the golden triangle. This opens up the upper airway so the tongue base can't fall backwards to block the windpipe. This is my surgical procedure. There's no algorithm; just the complete operation.

Fujita's result of his UPPP operation for OSA was evaluated 6 weeks after surgery using sleep studies. Great balls of fire! There were good short-term results with an overall reduction of RDI of 50%. There was improvement in snoring, and excessive daytime sleepiness. Again, temporary! Unfortunately, long term improvement was illusory. All the conditions returned. However, the results were considered positive enough to suggest a 6 hospital medical center study. Again, 50% improvement, temporary in nature. What's all the hullabaloo. The usual scientific double talk "let's improve the success rate by using a more refined patient selection criterion."

I modified the surgery to include the tongue base and epiglottis. The standard, UPPP was destined to become the number one surgery for OSA in the world.

The entire operation starts with a temporary tracheostomy. This hole in the neck is carried out using IV sedation and lots of local anesthesic xylocaine mixed with epinephrine. A curved endotracheal tube is placed and general anesthesia given. The upper airway is very fragile in OSA patients and deaths have been reported frequently. All patients undergo tracheotomy when risks are explained. Pre and post operative death is too horrible to contemplate.

The standard UPPP operation is continued. My approach to the tongue base is a controlled accurate removal. The technical advice for tongue base removal was shared by Doctor Tucker Woodson of the Medical College of Wisconsin. He arrived in Milwaukee after I finished by residency in 1969. He was most helpful in describing a perfect wedding cake slice. It resembled a piece of apple pie. He suggested anchoring the tongue with huge 2-0 ethicron suture. The line could support landing a shark. First, the sutures were pulled hard to lift the tongue upwards and tight toward the operating room light. A horizontal laser cut was made half-way up the tongue. The cutting cautery penetrated the hard, mucosal part of the tongue. Mayo scissors were used for a Lizzie Borden type incision connecting the deep tongue with the laser and cutting cautery cuts. This upward thrust with the scissors was directed toward the toes. It would bleed like stink for a few moments. This was the basic 2x2x4 cm piece of tongue base removal. No sutures were used to stop bleeding because vaginal packing pressure worked well. The tongue vessels retracted into the tongue substance.

The epiglottis covered the wind pipe and cookie-bite pieces of cartilage removed with an adenoid punch.

The reconstruction of the tissues in the tonsillar area produced a taut back wall of the pharynx. A small laser cut relaxed the tissue.

Fujita's UPPP operation is the most common operation for OSA. The long-term results are rather poor. Non-documented locker room gossip pegs the cure rate for mild OSA at 40%. The cure rate for moderate to severe OSA is basically zilch. Some dreamers place it at 20%. Many Universities do not operate on severe patients. They recommend CPAP. Using my technique Errigh La Boo, The Three Amigo's, and the Magnificent Seven are cured. My overall cure rate is 85% for mod-severe OSA long-term. It approaches 100% for less severe cases. It's the sinuses that are key. The ethmoid sinus operation combined with my modified UPPP affects the cure. As surely as Tinkers to Evers to Chance completed the double-play.

Other physicians have added breaking the facial bones including maxilla and mandible. Reconstruction includes moving teeth into normal occlusion. Also the neck bone (hyoid) has been assaulted. There's nothing I can add.

CHAPTER 21

The Full Monty – Part II

The Total Ethmoid Operation

Drs. May and Chaiken of the Shadyside staff
Teaching use of binocular operating microscope championed by Wolfgang Draf
Sitting down and using a two-handed technique
Doesn't tax my physique
Binocular vision makes the anatomy clear
Magnified images illustrates the tissues near
Blakesley instruments operate where ethmoid tissues lie
It's an easy as Mom's apple pie

The total ethmoid operation using the operating microscope was championed by Dr. Draf from Germany. The procedure was taught to me by Drs. Mark May and Barry Chaiken at the University of Pittsburg, Shadyside Hospital in 1996. The operating scope used a zenon fiber optic system of lighting of 1 million lucs. The brightness and clarity of this modified scope was incredible. Both hands were free to operate (Figs 10-13) in a 3-dimensional setting. This new view added depth perception to forestall any complicated anatomy in the ethmoid sinus; an inadvertent error could be assessed and corrected immediately. The microscope was modified by Zeiss and used for many years to the present.

The total ethmoidectomy operation was completed in the second day. There was removal of the vaginal packing, carefully checking for bleeding and general anesthesia given through the tracheotomy tube of day 1.

The bus picked me up at 7 AM for the trip to Shadyside Hospital. The ethmoid sinus CT scans are placed in the operating rooms view box for easy identification (Figure 10).

After the intubation, the binocular microscope is roled into place; the eyes are padded to protect the retina from the bright illumination of 1 million lucs (Figs 11, 12). Both hands are free to operate the scope, and use both hands for holding instruments or suctioning blood. The crystal clarity and brightness of the zenon system is like the sun rising above the Grand Canyon at day break.

This new technology with the added depth of perception made the operation safer. The anatomy of the ethmoid sinus, pre and post operatively allowed any inadvertent error to be identified and correctly immediately. The removal of the ethmoid cells and ostiomeal complex are seen in Figure 13.

The Full Monty is completed the next day. Nasal packing is removed under IV sedation (Deprovan) and the nasal packing removed with a nasal speculum and bayonet forceps. The temporary trach tube is replaced with a new, larger bore. The ethmoidectomy provides a decrease in the mast cell population. This is what I do! The results are quite satisfactory for my patients.

Fig 10

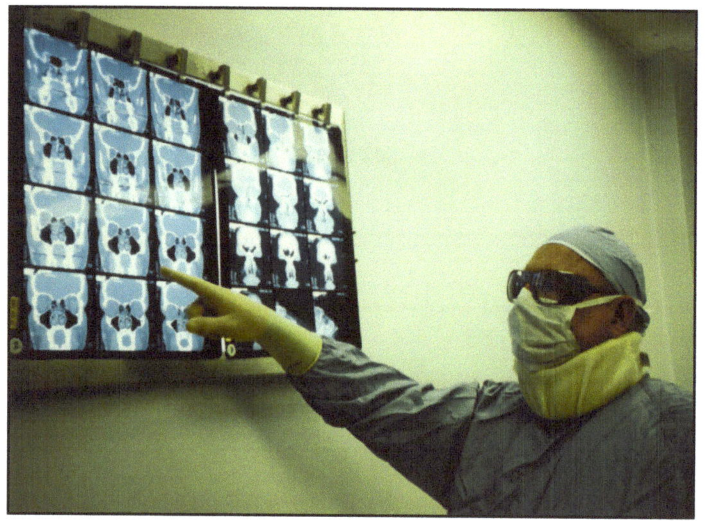

The total ethmoid operation
Ethmoid CT Scan on viewbox in operating room
Sinuses examined before and during surgery

Fig 11

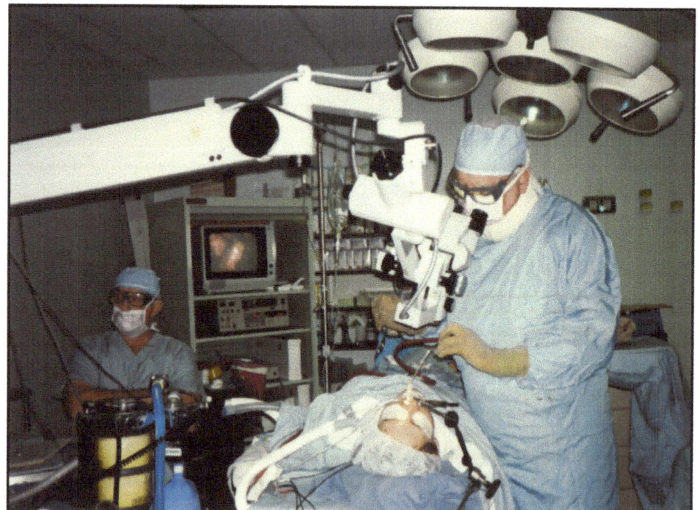

The total ethmoid operation
General Anesthesia
Operating microscope in place
Eye pads in place; both hands free
Anesthesiologist testing his eyes

Fig 12

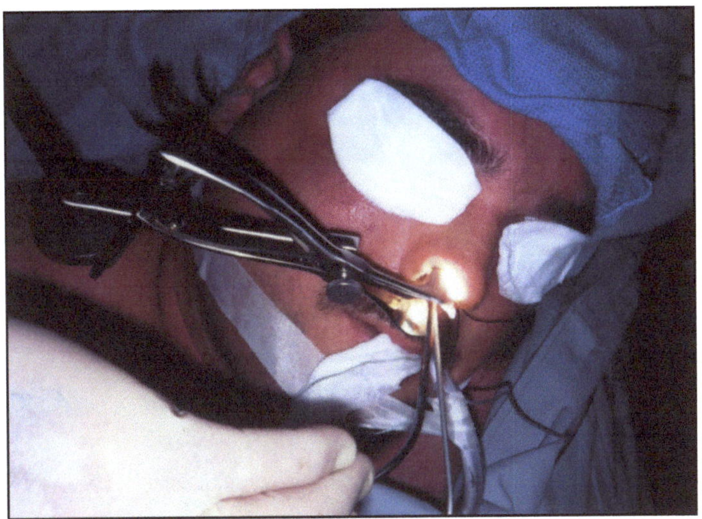

<u>The total ethmoid operation</u>
General Anesthesia
Self retaining nasal speculum in place
Eye pads on place
Beam of light from operating microscope

Fig 13

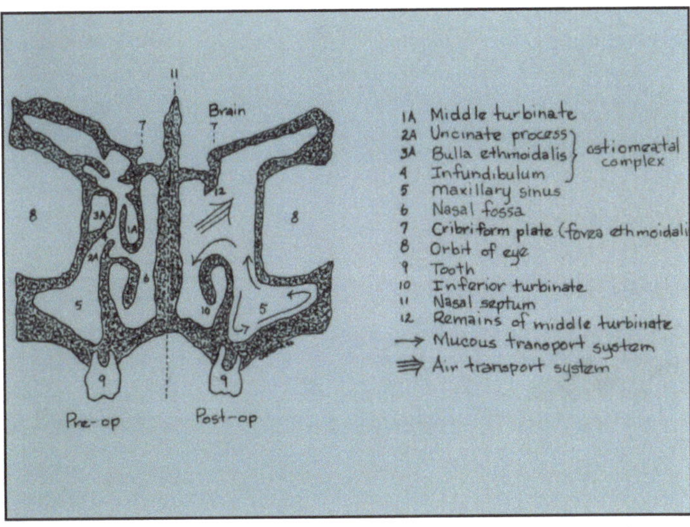

The total ethmoid operation. Ethmoid cells removed.
Ostiomeatal structures removed.
Pre and post OP views of total ethmoidectomy.
from Snore or Roar, 1996

CHAPTER 22

The Magnificent Seven (Interviews)
The Seven Samurai

Case Number 1	James Friday
Case Number 2	Joe Petrone
Case Number 3	Bill Strouse
Case Number 4	Joan Peters
Case Number 5	Mike Manichak
Case Number 6	Jefferson Hahn
Case Number 7	H. Burton

CHAPTER 23

James Friday

RR2 Box 354
Woodland PA 16881
814 857-7050

Case Number 1

James Friday and his wife Agnes (see photo's) were originally seen 7/13/00 in the Philipsburg office. Chronic fatigue, fragmented sleep, gasping at night and years of sinusitis with Nasal Obstruction contributed to snoring with OSA. A sleep study at the nearby Clearfield hospital by a sleep apnea group showed and RDI of 45 with an oxygen saturation of 72%. He wore CPAP for 2 months because of facial discomfort and claustrophobia. His RDI was 20 with CPAP. There was obesity and high blood pressure. These are ingrediants in the pathway to the metabolic syndrome zone. There was was facial skeletal deformily with and underdeveloped mandible. The Full Monty was done 8/2000. Elevated blood pressure returned to normal. The earliest clinical responses are the disappearance of snoring and sleep-disorder breathing. Follow up sleep study 5/8/01 showed no apneas, but hypopnea's present gave an RDI of 16 with a mean oxygen saturation of 95%. He did not use CPAP again.

Agnes worked in my office as a medical secretary for years observing pre and post-operative sleep apnea patients. Their daughter Dawn took over after they retired to Florida. Kim Yaple took over after Dawn was married and expecting.

Jim and Agnes were reinterviewed 6/7/07 (see photo's). Almost 8 years post operative his weight is 280 lbs. His original weight was 350 lbs. Blood pressure remains normal without medication. He has developed arthritis which runs in the family and is associated with damp weather. Florida weather helps and he hikes 3 miles daily. Bug bites recently caused some type of immune sickness. The addition of blood clots in the legs required Coumadin for 3 months. I wonder if this is an example for a cytokine storm. More about cytokines later.

Dawn has allergies and snores. She has two daughters. One is post op T & A and the other has allergies and asthma

He does not snore, feels great and enjoys life.

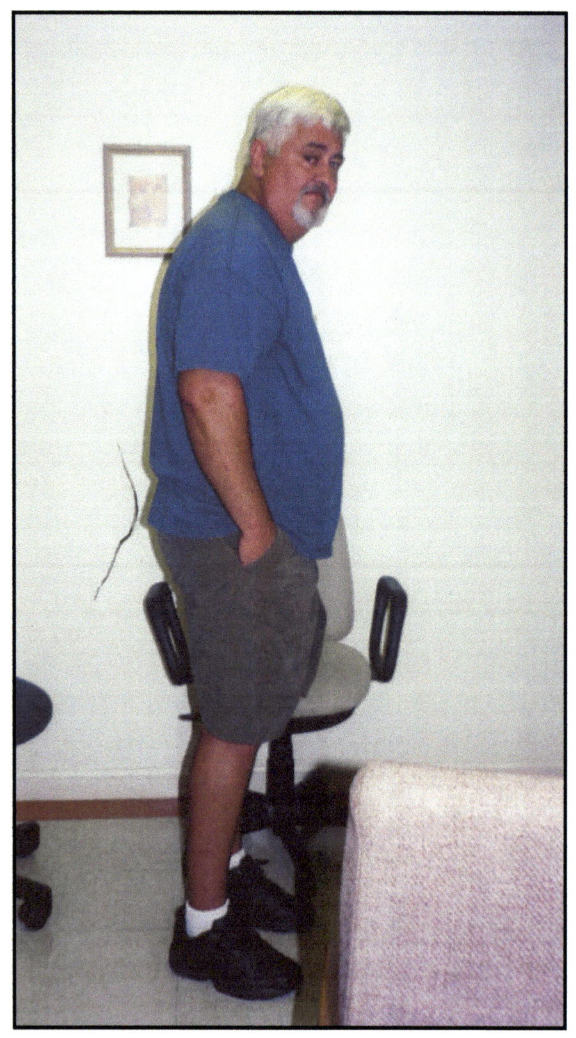
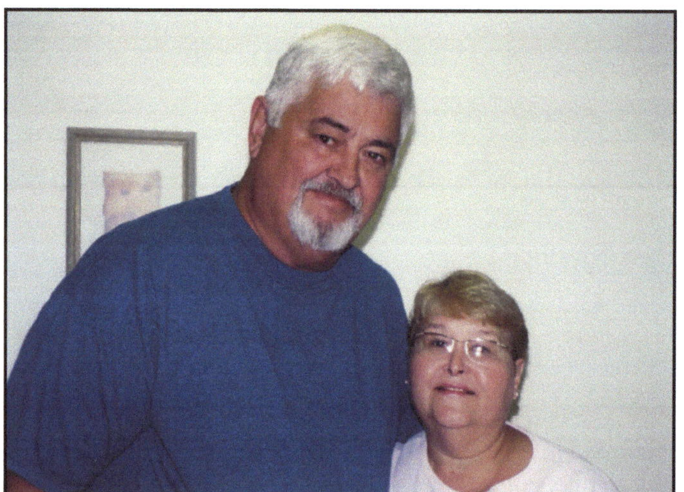
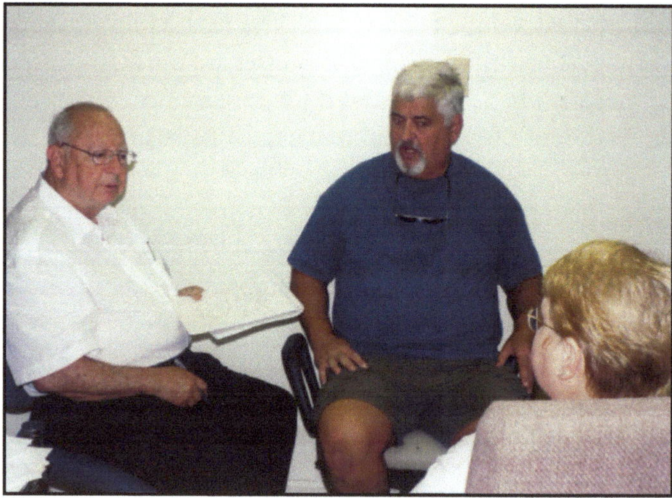

CHAPTER 24

Joseph Petrone

18 Evertum Circle
Plymouth Meeting PA
19462
610-275-9373

Case Number 2

Seen on 5/20/03 with the chief complaint of almost falling asleep driving. Nodding off at a light or falling asleep while talking or extreme forgetfulness is also associated with severe sleep apnea. I've had other patients (not Joe) flip their rigs, or have car accidents on their way to my office. This disease is dangerous. Traffic accidents from falling asleep is common. Traffic is stopped and backed up for miles. The helicopters are called. These buzzards circle the sky and drop down to pick up the bodies. Sleep apnea is much more than chopped liver.

Of interest, Joe's allergic to a variety of antigens and was treated medically for years. He was always a mouth breather and the CT scan of the ethmoids showed sclerosis. Ethmoid tissue removal only showed mast cells. It's a burnt out ethmoid cellular system. The cells were replaced by calcium salts.

His CPAP experience was brief. He has a severe overbite and the mask didn't fit well; also claustrophic. His RDI was 83.7 11/02 at Clearfield hospital. Post-op on 6/05 it was 7.0 His post-operative oxygen LSAT/% lose to 77 and the mean oxygen averaged 92. Because of facial overbite, he sleeps with his head propped up.

On 6/7/07 Joe was reinterviewed (see photo's) He's over 4 years post-operatively and doing quite well. His diabetes has not changed—still on glucophage. His restless leg syndrome is unchanged. His B.P. is usually normal but occasionally needs high B.P. meds. His cholesterol is normal now; he takes Lipitor. He does not snore or have sleep-disordered breathing. His fatigue and sleepiness have disappeared.

Family history shows that heart disease and high blood pressure affect his father. His mother has allergies and chronic mouth breathing. She's got lots of cholesterol and underwent coronary bye-pass surgery. His two children, boys; only one, the eldest, has allergies.

He is very grateful for his results, and offers his address and phone number if you seek advice.

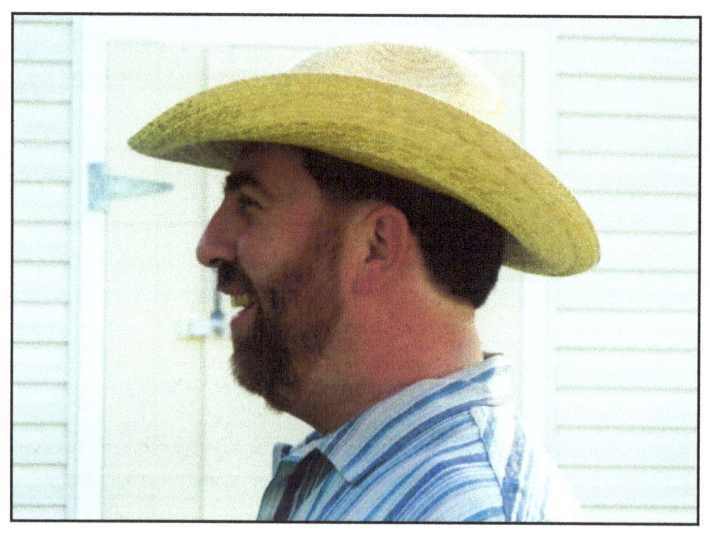

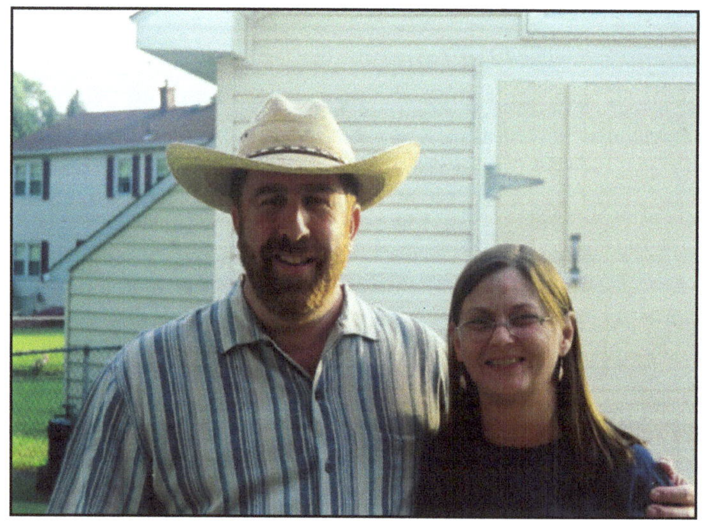

CHAPTER 25

William Strouse

2290 Trumbaursville Road
Quakertown PA 18951
215 538-7291

Case Number 3

Bill Strouse was seen at the office on 9/26/02. He was a trucker for Conway Trucking from Ann Arbor, Michigan. A sleep study had been ordered at North Penn Sleep Center. It showed an RDI of 32 and oxygen saturation to 74%. Restless Leg Syndrome (RDS) or Periodic Limb Movement Syndrome (PLMS) was prominent. He would wake up totally exhausted and almost fell asleep driving. CPAP was ordered and used intermittently for three months. Claustrophia caused Bill to rip it off; he headed for Philipsburg.

His sleep pattern was similar to my own OSA. Extreme drowsiness is frequent; falling asleep anywhere anytime is inappriate. Though it involves some loss of muscle control, its sleep apnea. I had sleep paralysis of my body while awakening from sleep. Just didn't panic and it disappeared shortly. Vivid, colour dreams are hypogogic hallucinations. Again they disappeared shortly. Though thought to be associated with narcolepsy, my belief is sleep apnea is the cause. Bill had some of these findings which is related to me in 5% of the cases. The ethmoidectomy, or "Full Monty" seems to eliminate these dream-like states. It may all be caused by the hormones produced in mast cells.

The Full Monty was performed 10/10/02. Six months later, a repeat sleep study at North Penn confirmed an overall RDI of 2 and a post operative mean oxygen level of 92%.

He was interviewed on 7/13/07 (see photo's) He feels great. No dreams, snoring, daytime sleepiness. Jumpy legs have disappeared and he gets a normal nights sleep. He sleeps 6 hours, and wakes up refreshed. He is allergic, on shots. BP is normal without medication. He has developed thyroid dysfunction requiring synthroid. One brother in good health except asthma, food and milk allergies as a child.

I remember meeting Bill at 3 AM at the local Exxon station in Philipsburg, post-op. Examined him at the office. He works at night to make a living. Why should he lose the bucks—food on the table comes first. What else could I do?

Bill is happy to answer your questions.

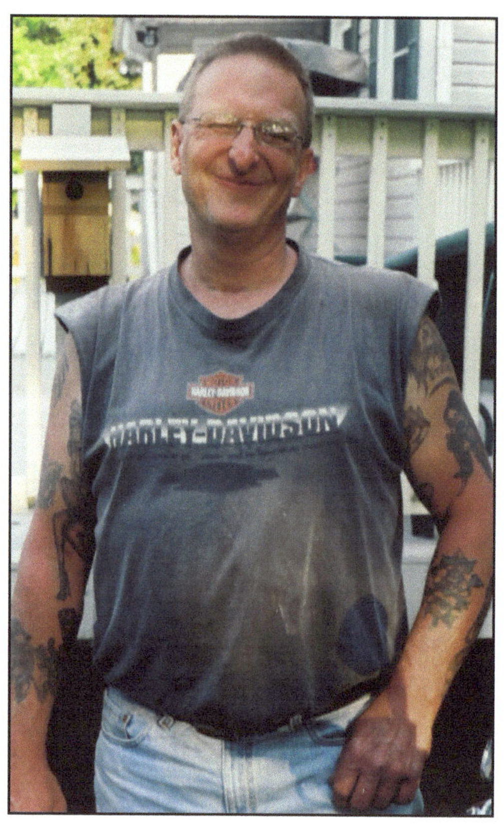

7/13/07
Bill Strouse

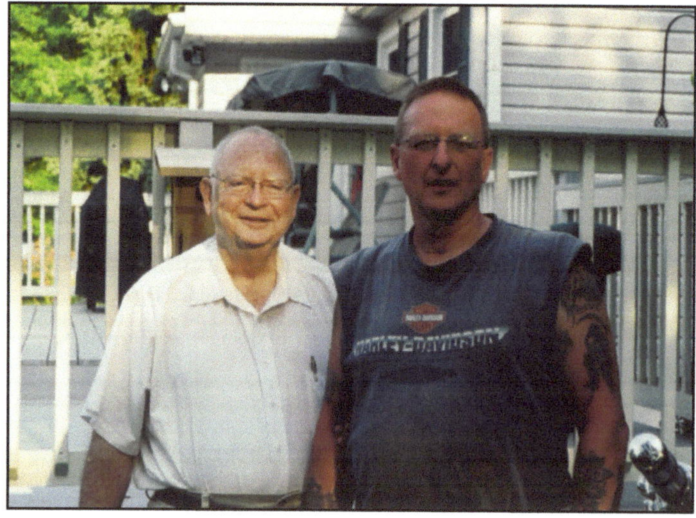

Dr. Newberg and Mr. Strouse

CHAPTER 26

Joan Peters

6850 Philipsburg/Bigler Hwy
West Decator PA
16878
814 342 0934

Case Number 4

Joan Peters was originally seen 6/16/07 in the office. She wore a CPAP faithfully for eight years but her OSA was worsening. Her memory dimished and she became forgetful. She had a sleep study 7/5/03 and the sleep specialist reported severe OSA with an RDI of 17 but an oxygen to 68%. This was compatible with her history of loud snoring, frequent arousals and significant weight gain. He never said or indicated it was done with CPAP. She had the Full Monty on 7/14/03. Of interest, she had psoariasis on her elbows and body pre-op. She was one of two OSA patients with psoriasis that cleared up after surgery. This is consistent with psoariasis as a immune-mediated disorder. T cells produce cytokines via the ethmoid system—the processing of an unknown antigen activates the T cell to migrate to the skin and trigger release of the cytokines (eg interferon) which causes the inflammation and rapid production of more T-cells and cytokines. More of this interesting aspect later. My theory of sleep apnea as a product of molecular biology fits nicely with allied immune diseases.

A repeat sleep study at Clearfield hospital post-operatively on 10/04, approximately 1½ years later shows only intermittent snoring without any apneas or hypopneas. She felt well rested. Her RDI was normal and the average mean oxygen level was 93%. Stages 1, 2 and 3 including REM were normal. No evidence of OSA. CPAP had been discarded after surgery. I smoked another one. I suppose one could use it as a fish tank pump. She moved it from the dresser drawer into the basement—next to the fish tank. The snoring and sleep apnea are gone.

She was interviewed on 6/29/07 (see photos) approximately 4 years after surgery. Her memory is better. No residuals of sleep apnea but her weight is up to 189 today (235 pre-op) She has no evidence of psoariasis. She stopped her allergy shots—she feels her allergies improved. Her blood pressure used to fluctuate—it's normal and stable. Her arthritis is stable. She takes Lipitor for high cholesterol. She walks 5 miles in the morning to get a paper; she's upset by watching a black bear destroy her bird feeders.

She has 3 children without signs or symptoms of OSA. Likewise, 1 brother and 1 sister do not have OSA.

She is very happy to speak to you re OSA.

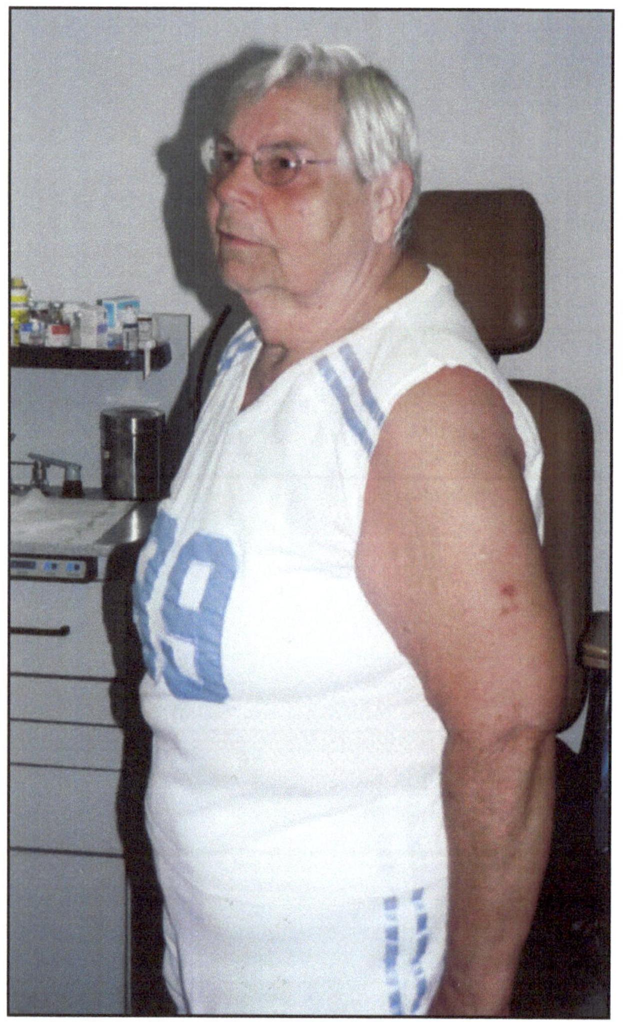

Joan Peters

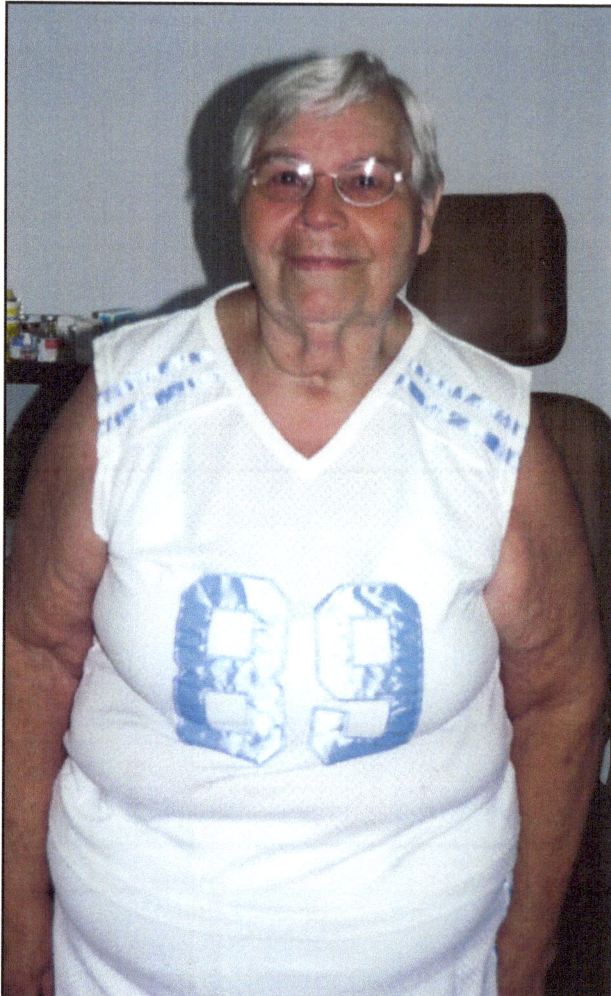

Joan Peters

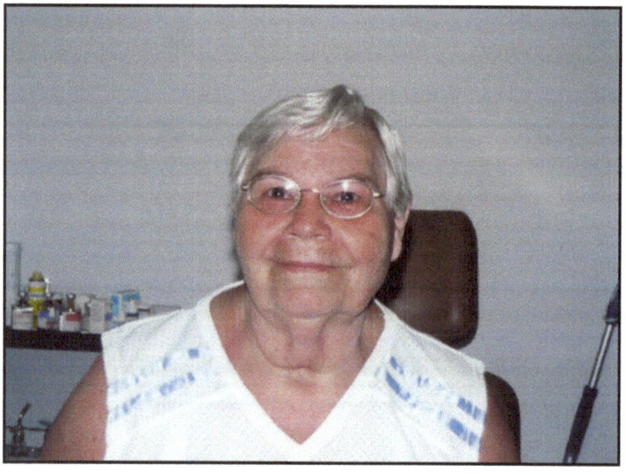

Joan Peters

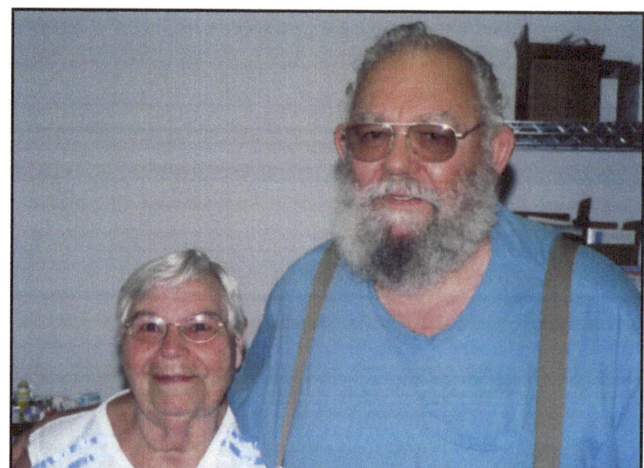

Joan and Calvin (husband) Peters

CHAPTER 27

Mike Mandichak

Home 304 Forest Dr
Ebensburg PA 15931
814 472-5031

Mid's Homemade Candy
Business 3135 New Germany Rd
Ebensburg PA 15931

814 472-5031
Store 814 472-6546 or
800 741-3951

Case Number 5

Mike Mandichak, the Candy Man, was first seen in the office 3/9/04. Mike makes and sells delicious chocolates His first documented sleep study at the University of Pittsburg Medical Center in 1998 showed an AHI of 90 and an oxygen saturation of 42%. This prompted an immediate CPAP. He could drift off and sleep anywhere, anytime. The sleep study shows mainly stage 1 and 2 sleep. This light sleep state is increased in OSA. Stages 3 and 4 brain waves are of the restorative deep sleep pattern. They are absent frequently Random eye movements (REM) sleep is usually disturbed from normal. The brain in OSA patients does not pass through the normal stages of dozing and deep sleep but goes in and out of REM sleep. The lack of deep sleep leads to a "catch up" period during the day, hence EDS. Dreams are common and catoplexy, such as head bobbing, are common. Sleep paralysis and hypogogic hallucinations are REM symptoms. The relationship between OSA, and REM symptoms is thought to be an autoimmune disease. Certain variations in T cells and the hormone neurotrophin produced in mast cells is the suspected autoimmune protein affected the neuron in the brain.

I first saw Mike in the office on 3/9/04. He wasn't doing well with CPAP after 4 years. Mike had hypogogic and hallucinogenic dreams with CPAP. His history suggested allergies though medications didn't help.

His physical started by measuring a size 22 inch neck. A deviated septum, ethmoid disease and soft, flabby throat tissues were obvious.

He underwent the Full Monty 3/04 and did well post operatively. He was reevaluated at the University of Pittsburg 5/05 over 1 year later. His symptoms of OSA resolved completely with denial of snoring, witnessed apnea and daytime sleepiness. Sleep study showed a few obstructive apneas/hypopneas with and RDI of 17. Mean oxygen saturation at night was 92%. The follow up pattern of sleep studies shows a residual of mild OSA. The clinical improvement, once started, gathers steam.

Mike and the missus, Mildred, (see photo's) were reinterviewed on 6/28/07. She doesn't hear any snoring and his breathing while asleep is normal. She wonders if he is alive.

In the 4 year post-op period his weight went from 300 to 245 today. His BP, cholesterol and blood sugar have not changed. He received allergy shots from 1956-62. He was retested and is on densenitization today.

Family history shows a brother with no OSA or allergies. A daughter age 15 started with mild spring pollen allergies only. Two son's have no allergies but snore. There is no history of asthma or obesity

Mike is symptom—free. He would be happy to share his experiences with you. CPAP remains locked-up in the basement.

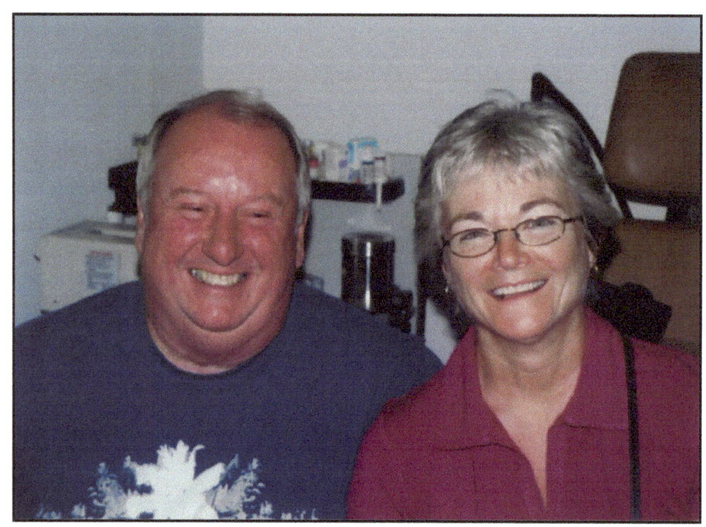

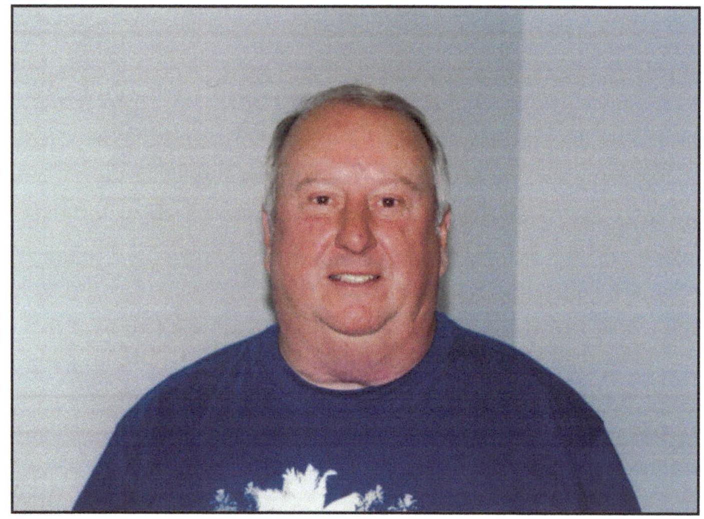

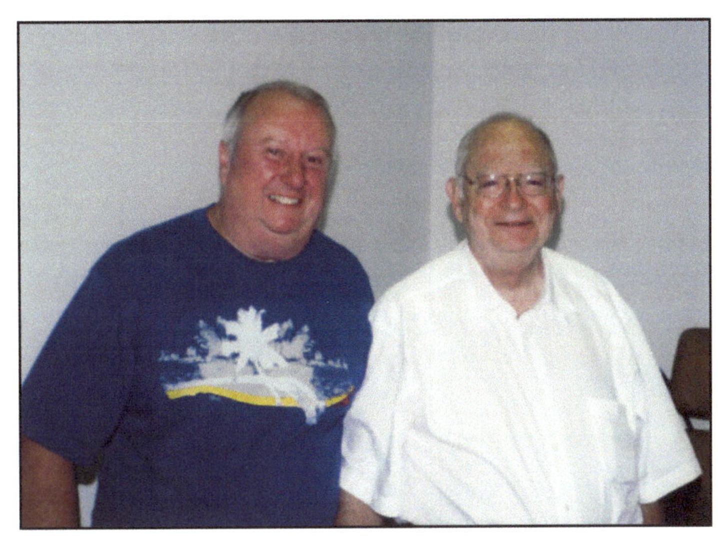

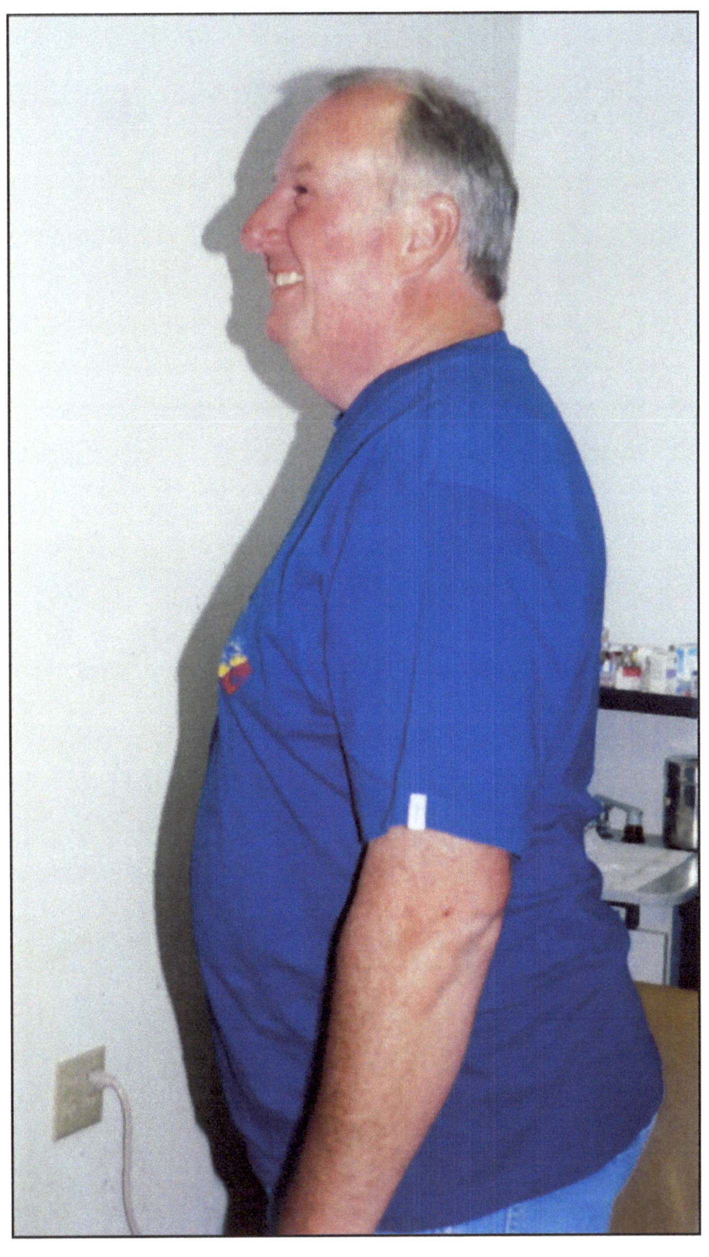

CHAPTER 28

Jeff Hahn

8 North Second St
Apt 8
Phillipsburg PA 16866
814 359 6478

Case Number 6

Jeff was a trucker. He was first seen in the office 4/6/04 for extreme somnolence. Can fall asleep anywhere, anytime. Neck size 25 and weight 350 lbs. Over 30 lbs since age 16. On 22 nasal oxygen 24 hrs/day for 1 year and wheelchair bound. On CPAP for 1 month only because of claustrophobia (a smothering effect) Sleep study at State College shows an RDI of 61 and a oxygen to 51%. He had impending respiratory failure. He had high B.P. and diabetes on insulin. He underwent to Full Monty 5/04. His BP returned to normal post-op. When reinterviewed 6/28/07, his diabetes was normal. No medications of any kind for diabetes.

A repeat sleep study et West Penn hospital center for Sleep Disorders on 7/14/05. This is 14 months post op. There was zero (zilch) sleep-disordered-breathing events. His oxygen was markedly improved and the SpO_2 at 94% was good.

His pulm. function tests show mild obst. lung defect (2/18/04).

He was interviewed 6/28/07 (see photo's.)-3 years post-op. He has clinically lost all stigmata of the Pickwickian syndrome. Dickens wrote the selected Pickwick papers and fat Joe described the poster boy for the future Pickwickian syndrome. His weight to fell 185 and today weighs 220 lbs.

He was recently operated for a ruptured disc but has stenosis of the spine. He quit insulin and all meds; the blood sugars are normal.

He walks the streets of Phillipsburg daily for about 3 miles. He doesn't use oxygen or CPAP. He is atopic and is undergoing desens.

He has no serious heart disease.

He is doing quite well and would consider it pleasure to discuss his condition.

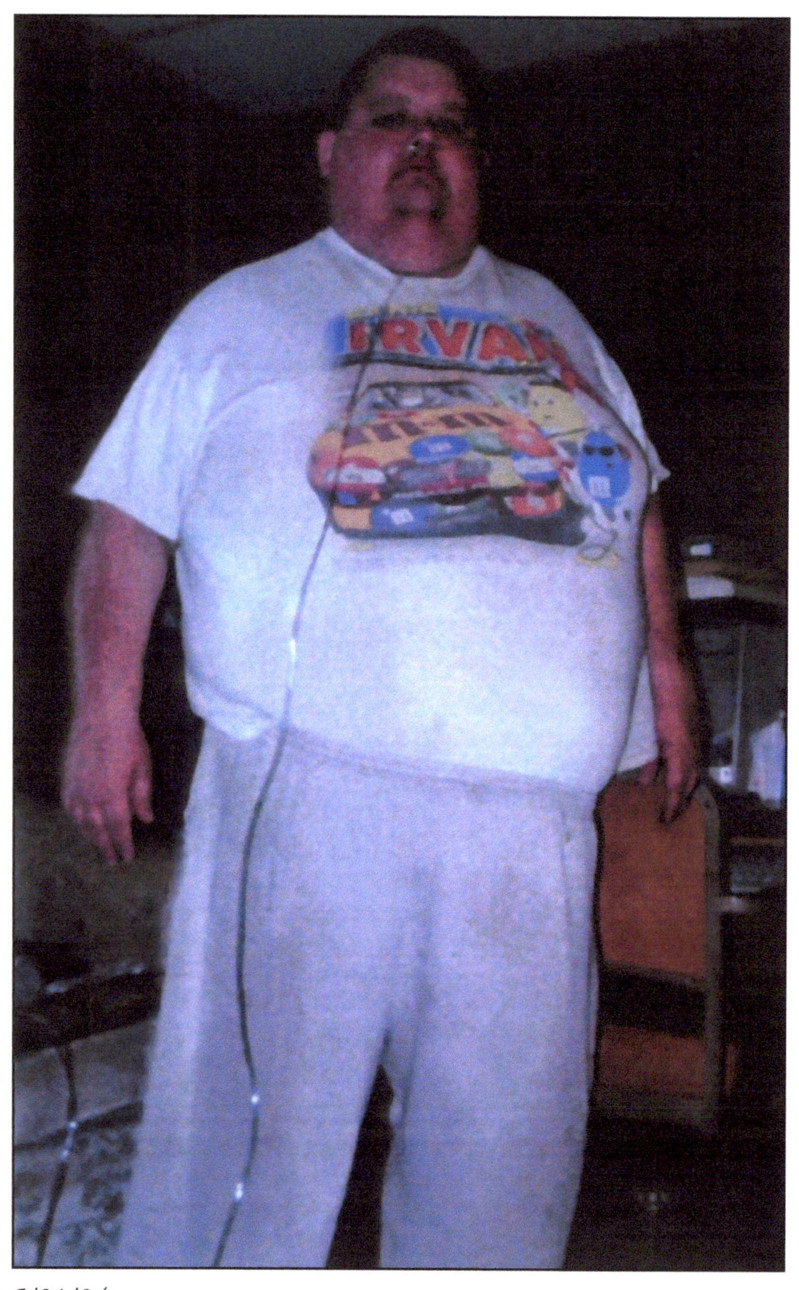

5/01/04 pre-op

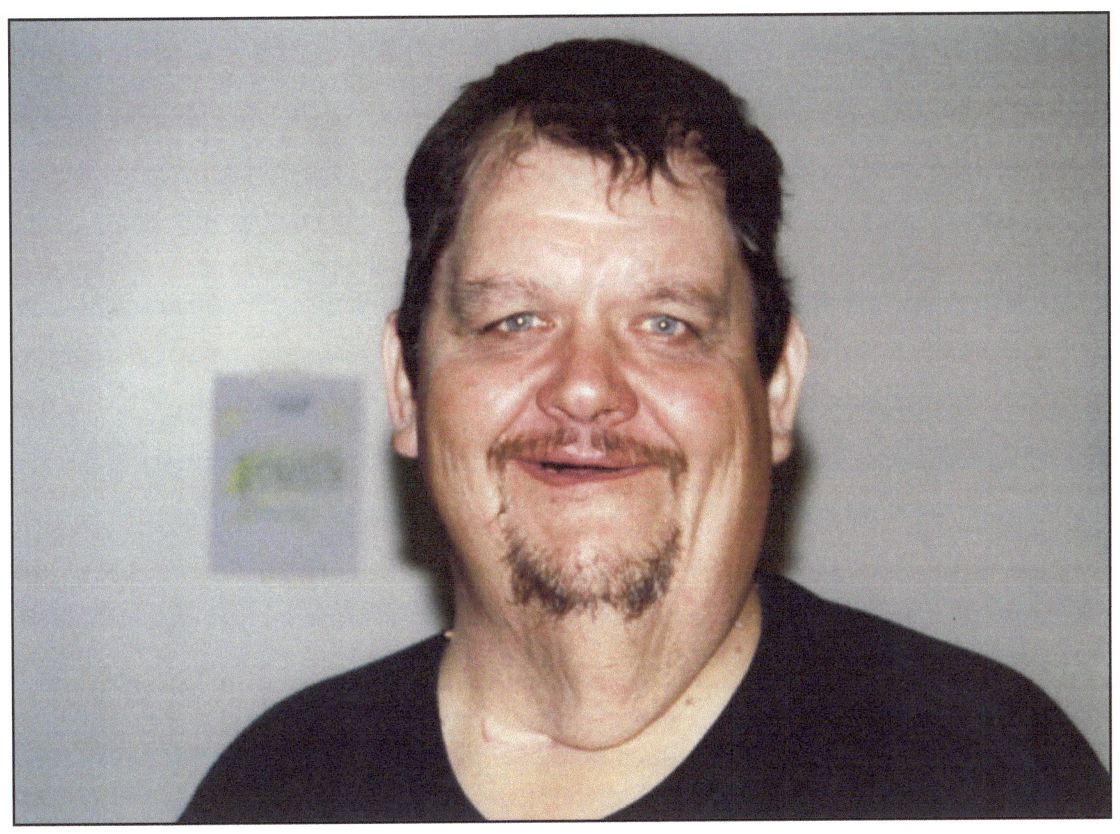

6/28/07 post-op

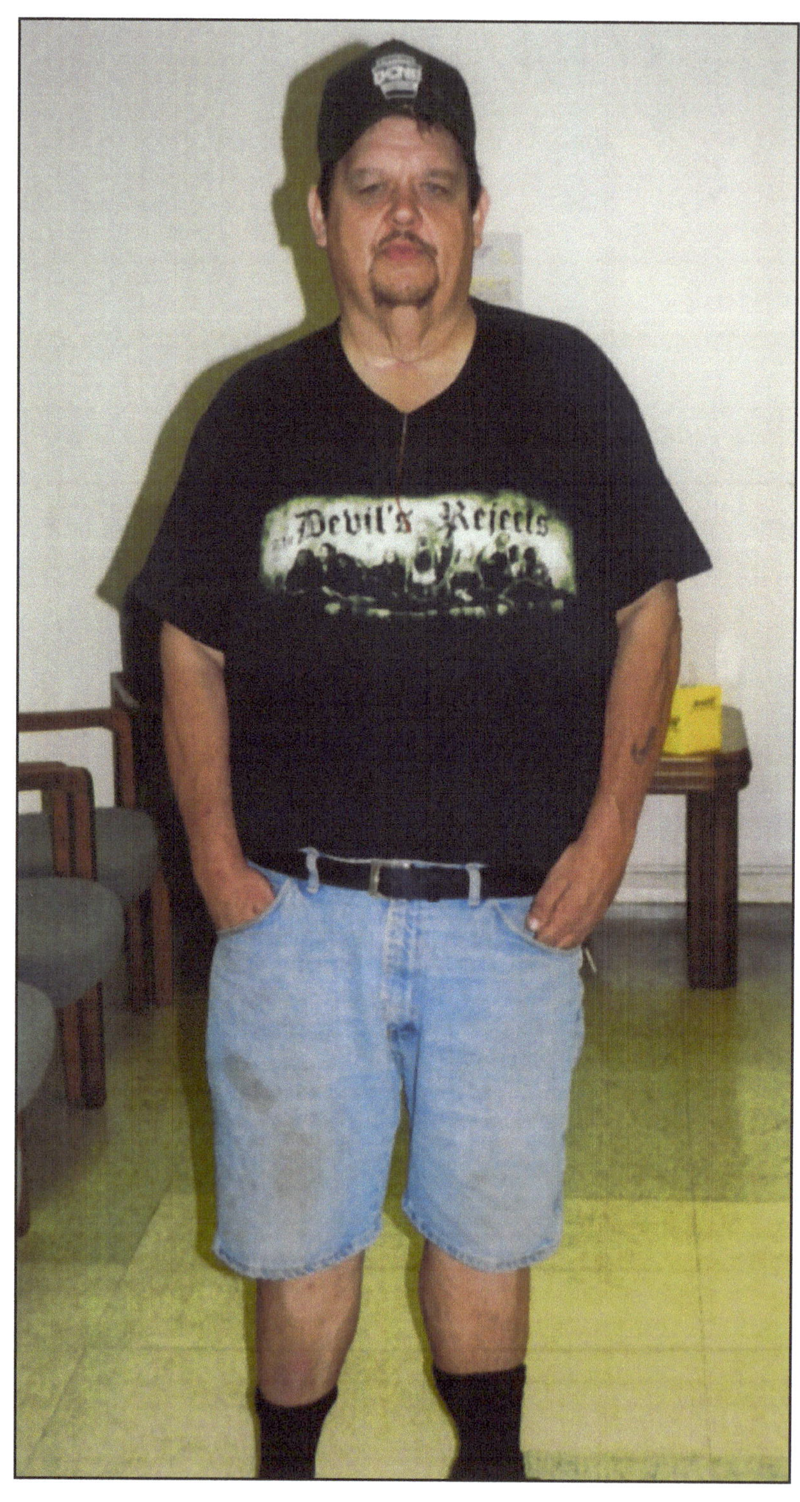

6/28/07 post-op

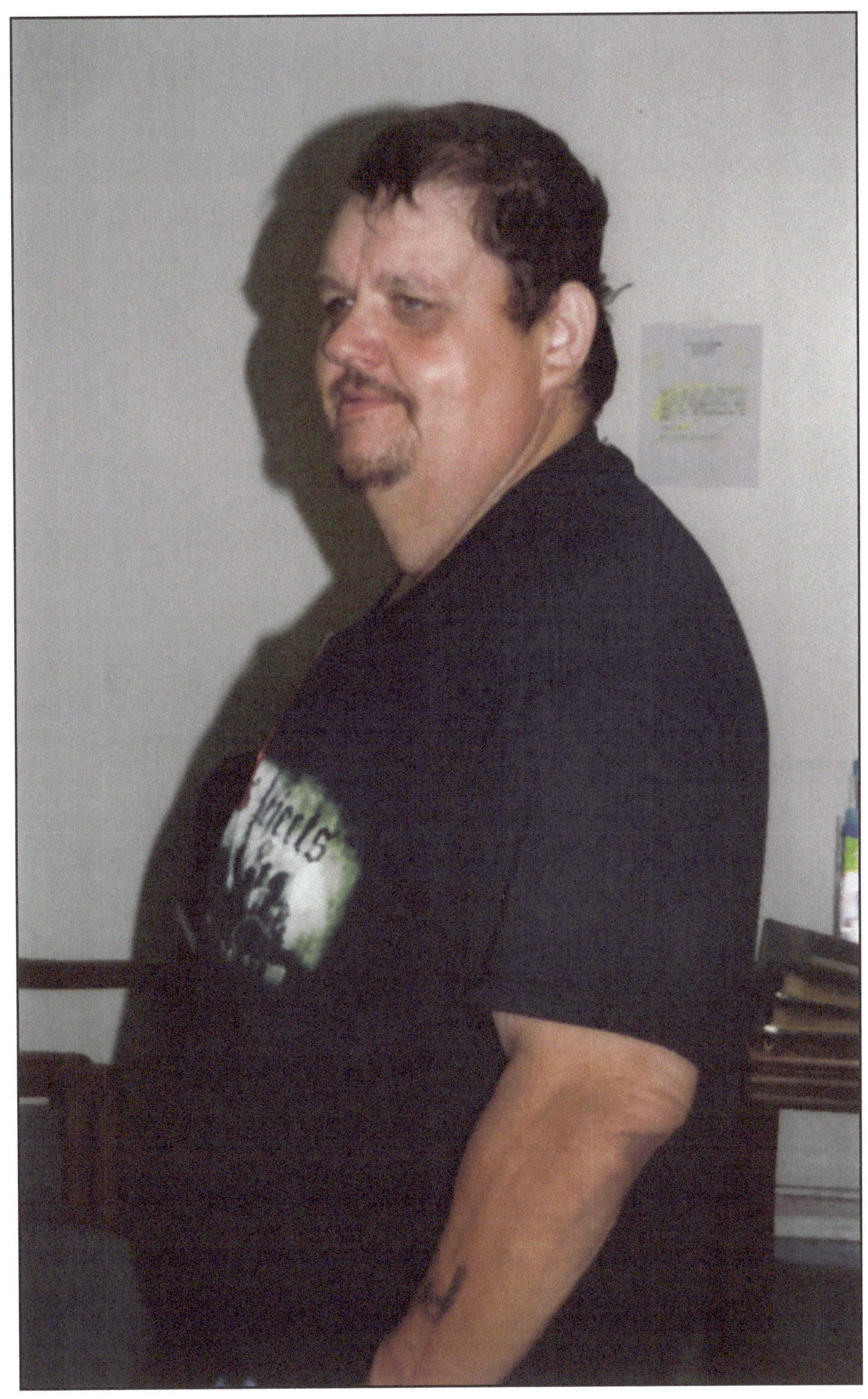

6/28/07 post-op

CHAPTER 29

Howard Burton

P.O. Box 12
123 West 5th St
Burnside PA 15721
814 845-2419

Case Number Six

First seen in the office 8/24/04. Blind from diabetes; high B.P.; Falls asleep sitting up, snores, restless sleep. XDS. takes insulin 50-60 u humologue. Has glaucoma and jumpy legs, wore CPAP 3 years, Bi PAP 2 years—no help at present

Sleep study at Indiana Regional Medical Center. RDI of 101; REM RDI of 69 non-REM of 109 SpO_2 61% Little Stages 3 & 4; stages 1 and 2 increased; REM decreased.

Surgery 9/04—the Full Monty By 12/7/04 B.P. was normal without medications no sleep disordered breathing; on allergy shots.

Repeat sleep study 3/14/05 at Clearfield hospital RDI of 41 with mean oxygen saturation of 95% No CPAP used since surgery; still has RLS; now alert and awake after 6 hrs sleep

Reinterviewed 6/28/07 (see photo's) over 2½ years post. op.

Blind from diabetes pre-op

Previously received 50-60 units Humalog

Now 8-10 units before eating and 20u Lente at night; stopped allergy shots.

Sa O_2 while sleeping 97-99%-tested at nursing home. Well, alert without depression and to receive a seeing eye dog for mobility. Markedly improved clinically

Two sisters, son daughter without OSA mild snoring at most—no sleep disorder noted by staff and pt is well rested and alert.

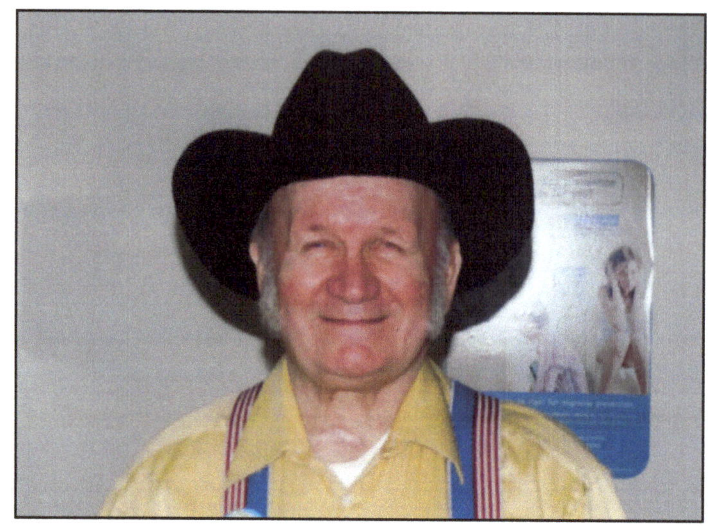
Howard Burton

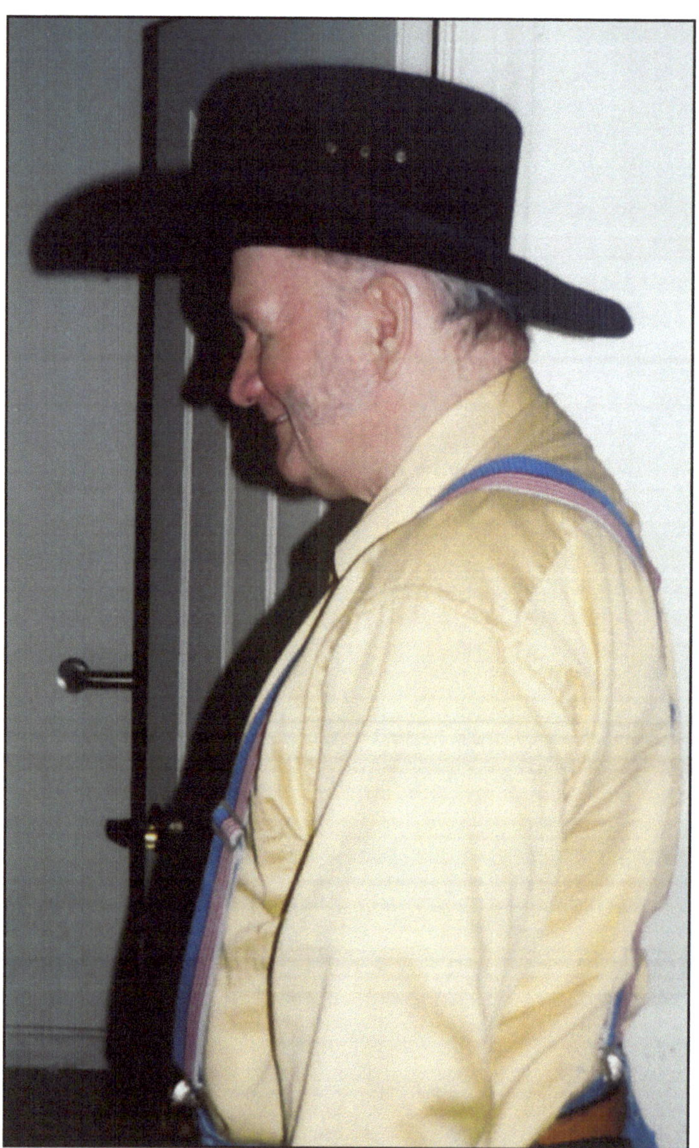
Howard Burton

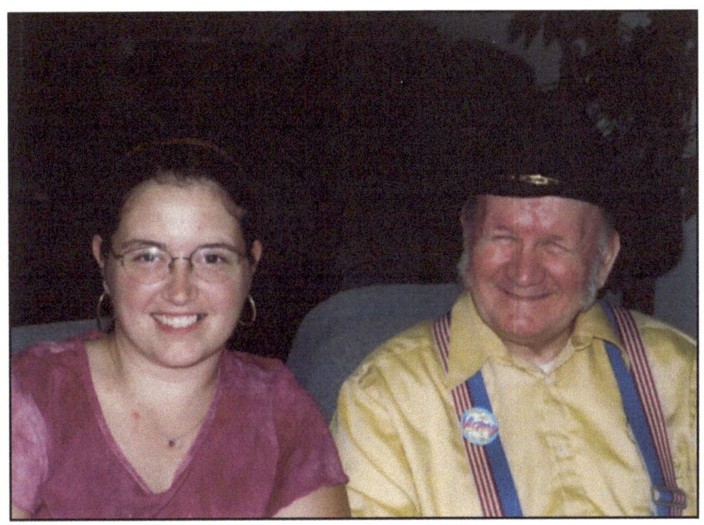

Howard Burton, care-giver

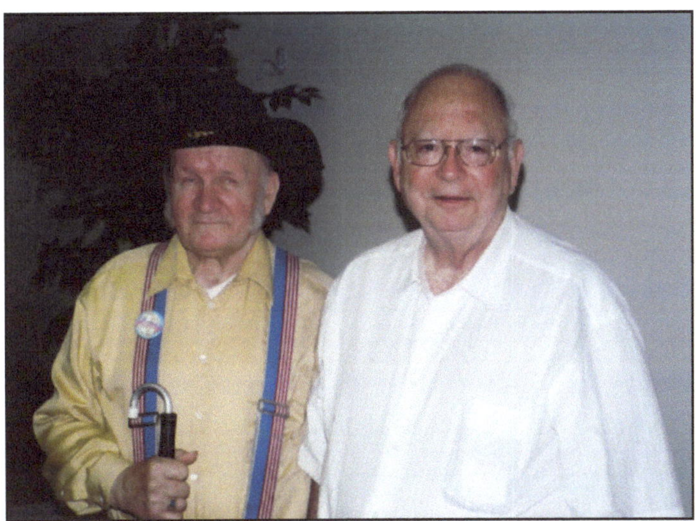

Howard Burton, Doctor Newberg

CHAPTER 30

Results of the Seven Samurai

Results of the Seven Samurai
Are not considered Chazarai
From 1980 onwards, OSA increased to a pandemic
The "how" and "why" of the metabolic syndrome are more than academic
Activated immune complexes are held together by ligands
They are reversible with the strength of a rubber band
The Full Monty cures OSA
Also returns the metabolic syndrome to normal in the US of A
The Full Monty works just fine
To decimate mast cells and the cytokine
RDI's can reach the sky
Returning to normal fills one with joy
Carrying the load of obesity
Raises the specter of eternal adversity
I feel the power of the Phoenix birds glory
That mystical bird makes one heck of a story
The cure of OSA resurrects the living dead
To an eternal life in Club Med

Starting in 2000, seven consecutive patients wearing CPAP for various lengths are time, and shown to suffer from moderate to severe OSA including the trappings of a variety of metabolic syndrome complications. Surgery was chosen for the study because criteria for cure would be observable to a lay person. The cure rate in the past, for these types of cases, approached zero. I wonder if CPAP was developed to treat OSA surgical failures. The patients were all reinterviewed for the book in the later part of 2007. They are very happy with the results having long-term cures. Mr. La Boo, operated in 1996 is eleven years, post-operative. They are appreciative to share their experience with anyone interested in their results. Since I'm the only surgeon using this innovative surgery, they would like to pass on the message.

Table 2 shows the mean RDI was 61.4; post-operative RDI was 12.0. The range of RDI was 17-101 pre-operatively and 0-41 post-operatively. The LSAT prior to surgery averaged 61%; post-surgery, it was 85.4%. Post-operative mean oxygen saturation was 93% (I think this is the most important number). The post-operative sleep study was performed an average of 27.5 months after surgery. To prevent any hanky-panky with the sleep study data, all sleep studies were done at sleep study centers in hospitals. I had no input in the choice of location but prefer West Penn or the University of Pittsburg sleep centers. All were read by board-certified sleep study physicians at the centers.

The response to clinical changes in the metabolic syndrome are in Table 3. The newest data in 2007 reflects further improvement in those disease. Joan Peters psoariasis never reappeared after surgery. The latest weights are given in the reinterview—confirmation can always be obtained from the patient. Even Restless Leg Syndrome all three cases.

The mean weight of the seven pre-op was 279 lbs; post-op 225 lbs. Some patients experience extreme weight loss. None had any weight reduction surgery . . . . like gastric by-pass Jeff Hahn, Pickwickian, started at 350-380 lbs, fell to 185 and is 220 at the interview 6/28/07.

The diabetic patients have all improved. Jeff Hahn no longer uses insulin and Howard Burton takes a greatly reduced doseage. The immune respones of mast cells in ethmoid tissue and skin testing in Table 4 shows good correlation.

Over 100 cases have been completed. The moderate to severe OSA patients have a cure rate of 85% long term with lesser severe cases approaching 100%.

Table 2. Seven Consecutive Moderate-Severe OSA Patients Using CPAP-Surgically: Treated 2000-2005

Patient No./Age Y, Sex	CPAP Duration mo.	Date of Surgery mo./y	RDI PSG/Date		LSAT/%		Mean SaO_2/% post-op
			Pre-op	Post-op	Pre-op	Post-op	
1/57/M	4	8/00 incl. septoplasty	45 (1/00)	16 (5/01)	72	86	95 (96% time > 90)
2/50/M	0.5	7/03 incl. tonsillectomy	83.7 (11/02)	7 (6/05)	60	77	92 (72% time > 90)
3/49 M	3	10/02 incl. septoplasty, tonsilectomy	32 (4/02)	2 (4/03)	74	87	92.3 (98% time > 90)
4/69/F	96	7/14/03 incl. tonsils	17 (7/03)	0 (10/04)	68	87	93 (98% time > 90)
5/51/M	72	3/04 incl. septoplastly	90 (5/98)	17.6 (6/05)	42	84	93 (89% time > 90)
6/47/M	1	5/04	61 (2/04)	1 (6/05)	51	94	87-93 (placed on 2L Nasal O_2: 100% time > 90)
7/63/M	18	9/04 incl. septoplasty, tonsillectomy	101 (1/03)	41 (3/05)	61	83	95 (96% time > 90)

Note on Table 2

Abbreviations: RDI: Respiratory Distress Index; PSG: Polysomnography; CPAP: Continuous Positive Airway Pressure; LSAT: Lowest Oxygen Saturation; SaO_2: Mean Oxygen Saturation. All surgies include bilateral total ethmoidectomy, midline glossectomy, cranial epiglottectomy, and temporary tracheostomy. Additional surgeries (indicated) include septoplasty and/or tonsillectomy.

Patient 2 had severe Max/Mand Skeletal Deformity and slept in High Fowler Position. Patient 6 showed Pickwickian symptoms. Pre-op, nasal O_2 7/24/365 days a year, wheelchair-bound, hypovent. and obst. lung disease by pul. fx. Post-op, IL Nasal O_2 per night, discarded CPAP and wheelchair, currently walks 5 miles/day.

Table 3. Metabolic and Restless Leg Syndrome in OSA Patients

Patient	Height (in.)	Weight (lbs.)		Blood Pressure		RLS		Diabetes Mellitus
		pre-op	post-op	pre-op	post-op	pre-op	post-op	
1	75	350	310	High	Normal	No	No	
2	70	200	180	High	Normal	No	No	Diet controlled; No change
3	68	200	212	High	Normal	Yes	No	
4	61	235	161	Normal	Normal	No	No	
5	70	300	270	Normal	Normal	No	No	
6	69	350	215	High	Normal	No	No	Humulin 70/30 to oral agent
7	70	222	184	High	Normal	Yes	Yes	No change in insulin

Table 4. Immune Responses in
Seven OSA Patients

Light Microscopy of Ethmoid Tissue Mast Cells (1-3+) or Sclerosis (s)			Skin Testing – Allergic Rhinitis Inhalant Allergens			
Patient	Right	Left	Pollens	Fungi	Mites	Dust
1	3+	3+	1+	2+	3+	3+
2	1+	1+	Pos.	Pos.	Pos.	Pos.
3	2+	2+	Pos.	Neg.	Pos.	Pos.
4	3+	3+	Pos.	Pos.	Pos.	Pos.
5	1+	1+	Pos.	Pos.	Pos.	Pos.
6	1+	1+	Pos.	Neg.	Pos.	Pos.
7	S	S	Pos.	Pos.	Pos.	Pos.

Table 2 lists pertinent pre and post-operative information in the surgery treated from 2000-2005. The date of surgery m/year. The "Full Monty" and total ethmoid operations

Table 3 Pre and post operative "Metabolic Syndrome" changes including Restless Leg Syndrome (RLS) Blood pressure, diabetes and weight

Table 4 The immune responses in tissue mast cells of the ethmoid. Also skin testing using inhalant and pollen antigen extracts

CHAPTER 31

The Medical License
Or
Easy Come, Easy Go

This last surgeon
Carry's an everlasting burden
I accuse the Medical Society
Acting the part of a childish deity
Research and innovation
Treated as a foreign notion
The universe had the Big Bang
The legal profession has a gang
It was Mike Nilfong
Acting like King Kong
Sham medical peer review
Doctors don't have a clue
Life liberty and the pursuit of happiness
The Medical Society ignores due process
The Medical Society perpetuates their nonsense
You lose your medical license
The medical politician and hospital administrator
Are ruthless intimidators
And when all is said and done
Your medical license is gone

The academic institutions in Baltimore are split into two factions. The John Hopkins Medical Centre and the University of Maryland are separated by a fish market, history and class. John Hopkins physicians always wear a leather patch on the sleeves of their jackets. Being from the Midwest, and having no academic credentials, I was relegated to a number of smaller hospitals and staffs. Sinai, Lutheran, Montgomery General and South Baltimore General (renamed Harbour) hospitals were mine. My medical education continued with continuing medical education (CME) credits from courses at the American Academy of Otolargngology. The teachings of Doctor David Austin in Chicago, before moving to Utah. He was an outstanding scientist research with world-class credentials in ear and mastoid surgery. The other was Doctor Thane Cody, President of the Academy and Chairman of the Ear, Nose, and Throat Department at the Mayo Clinic. They presented their theories and surgical results in the scientific literature. Their research in the chronic inflammatory disease of the mastoid bone and sinuses (ethmoid) showed profound effects on functions of the sinuses/mastoid. My results, gleaned from knowledge at the Academy were excellent.

My knock on the door came in 1977. The Last Surgeon (me) answered. A combined Blue Cross/Blue Shield taskforce would question my knowledge and procedures. It was a little more gross. The insurance company targeted those doctors it feels cost them too much money.

Working in cahoots with the State Peer Review Committee of Public Safety, BC/BS knew the expected findings and results. It didn't take long for the Attorney General to sit at the meeting table.

The peer review process has favored the status quo. In 1896, the disease rabies, was a certain killer. The bite of a rabid animal led to the painful demise. In the 1890's, a French chemist would isolate rabid tissue, weaken the immune agent (let's call it a virus) by air drying rabid brain tissue. Then a series of shots from the tissue to build up an immunity. In 1986, a ten year old girl exhibiting the first signs of rabies was injected with the new vaccine. She promptly died. The French Medical Society went ballistic! They called the chemist a murderer. They would remove his medical license if he possessed one. Incarceration sounded the proper punishment. Detentions would come later, in an enlightened twentieth century. He would have shared a cell with Doctor Kevorkian.

Treatments for rabies in the 1890's were poultices. These were soft substances of roots spread on cloth. They were moistened by the saliva from the dog bite. Also the poultice was heated and medicated with rabid dog urine. Yes, your Medical Society was at work. Of course, the chemist was Louis Pasteur and he cured rabies.

The statute is a permanent collection of State laws. Violation of the statute, as determined by a State Peer Review Committee means sanctions against the physician. The result is than many doctors have been targeted on frivolous or even made up evidence. A systemic corruption of the Medical Board has ruined many doctors' lives. The victim of a fraudulent peer review is judged by others who incur no expense or inconvenience. A final meal, the "doctors" last supper is served. The members have total immunity from any prosecution. Hundreds of thousands of dollars for defense will be spent. Temporary suspension of license upon appeal is rarely granted. Your name appears in the monthly journal under "Your Medical Society at work." And the State has the Chutzpah to raise fees to offset the cost to the State. Most doctors are innocent and suffer in silence. Where's the media? Where's a watchdog committee? The health care crisis will require a resolution. Defensive tests and a decrease in cutting edge surgeries will occur.

There is the presumption in the Peer Review process of impartiality. Due process, as a constitutional right, should be observed. Selection of the victim is neither impartial nor fair. I accuse BC/BS of abuse of power. Until insurance companies are removed from favoritism with the Board, this unholy alliance will fester. Also, insurance companies have their own investigatory bodies, and patients allegedly wronged, can always report their case directly to the Board.

Doctor Harold Sernaker placed a transplantable nerve blocker into a patient's back. The patient didn't do well. A complaint was filed. Gone!

Doctor Gerald Miller, Board Certified Ophthalmologist, did "too many cataracts," as reported in the Baltimore Sun. Gone!

Doctor Alan Greenberg practiced Neurology using holistic medicines. Tarred and feathered at Medical Society headquarters. Never seen again. Gone!

The modus operandi of the Medical Society and institutions is to reduce the freedoms of innovation. Christian Barnard received a two-year scholarship in cardiothoracic surgery at the University of Minnesota. He returned to the Groote Schuur Hospital in South Africa. In 1967, his first heart transplant was heard around the world. I am disappointed that the surgery didn't take place in Minnesota. What happened? Why not? We can be sure the internal dynamics of the hospital medical politicians and administrators will cover this up quite nicely. Thank you!

Jack Kevorkian was a public champion of a terminal patient's right to die. Physician assisted suicide struck terror in the community; or did it? The Doctor of Death had his license revoked. The choice of choking to death with allied findings in Amyotrophic Lateral Sclerosis should be a patient's choice.

In Milwaukee, John Just, a chest Surgeon, gave blood transfusions, and lots of them, to terminally ill cancer patients. The Veterans hospital was always short of blood for John's patients. One day, he gave 2 units of blood to a dying veteran. When he was still alive 24 hours later, and John had the garden hose ready, the patient cursed him out. He died in peace a few hours later. John became known as "John the Just." He was as screwy as Huey and Louie!

The first salvo from exceeding BC/BS guidelines were high lighted. BC/BS had hired flunkies to provide independent, unbiased testimony. A quick vote after scanning the records, and hearing pontification of the glorious peer review system. Whereas BC/BS covered costs from their subscribers, I paid my legal fees. There was the additional cost of medical experts and physicians willing to testify. The meter was running.

In 1977, my exposure to innovative ideas, and performing cutting edge technologies blew their minds. Their attitude was "we are the experts, and who are you to question us." The mastoid operation in chronic serous otitis media (CSOM) ticked them off. The community standard was the plastic pressure equalization tube (PET). This was the community standard, now and forever. And the half hour spent for a complete mastoidectomy with a facial recess approach blew their minds. The Peer Review Committee was anchored by Professor Blanchard of the University of Maryland. The rest of the committee was composed of Samuel Lumpkin, clinical Professor at John Hopkins and Anthony Hammond, instructor at Saint Agnes Hospital. Besides these three experts, one sickly looking Board Certified specialist was Stanley Blum, the obligatory Jew. They gave me lip service. Since my license is all I have, my defense was rooted in Marvin Ellin, a tough malpractice attorney. As he told me, "I was terminal and in the ICU."

It was my mentors that taught me the indications, procedures and techniques to the rescue. They have the moral courage to confront the Medical Society. Both Thane Cody of the Mayo Clinic and David Austin came to my defense. Actually, they were defending ideas taught at the Academy.

The complaints were manipulated to fit into the fraud statues. My lawyer pulled a Perry Mason. By the wall clock, my mastoidectomy with facial recess approach and tube insertion was completed in 30 minutes, start to finish. The Peer Review unit said it was a lesser procedure than a mastoidectomy. It should be billed at a lower rate. My two experts identified the surgery as a mastoidectomy, just as I described. For the first, and perhaps the only time, a doctor under sentence of death was reprieved. My father taught me the difference of opinion from a lie. My experts saved me. Otherwise, my work on OSA would be interrupted permanently.

Forced to accept a reprimand for five cases, anger set in. Three of the cases were about mastoids, and I wrote a scientific paper on mastoidectomy for chronic serous otitis using these three cases. It made me feel better.

The other two cases were chest x-rays on children with fever and cough. They had pneumonia on x-ray. The Peer Review Committee said chest x-rays are not necessary to diagnose pneumonia. You can make the decision.

The statute is a permanent collection of state laws. Il trovatore, the anvil chorus, is opera's background for the greatest "bing-bong" of all time. Michael Nifong changed the medical statutes. There's now a Fecal statute; whereby a fictitious crime fits somewhere. He got caught! Probably the odor. The Bupkis statute (where there's no crime to the Nth degree) and the "Gotcha" standard of one-up-man-ship. This meshugge was a Schlock Lawyer. This is a poorly made law with the appearance of abuse. This macher gave spielkes to the entire legal system. Imagine how doctors feel when they've been Nifonged. As my mother said, "Its Oy! Oy! Oy; doctors are not a play toy." Yes Mike Nifong, doctors are not chazarai. The Nifongs of the world are alive and well on Medical Society and hospital staffs. Beware the trumped up charges based on flimsy evidence; allegedly for political purposes.

And the legal State authorities have the chutzpah to charge a yearly fee to offset the cost of sham charges. Look no further than the 6 lambs from Duke University Lacrosse ready to be barbecued for Nifongs political ambitions. There's a breakdown in the moral conduct of the Medial Peer Review System. The "guilty physician of the month" from misinterpreted and forged evidence will destroy the system. Innovation may stop in order to be politically correct.

And the safeguards of our freedom are being eroded. Where's the press scrutinizing the Medical Society Nifongs. Many doctors who obtain a financial or political benefit by government fiat are happy. Doctor "No", the medical director of an HMO, never saw a necessary surgery. The violation of ethics, the crime of moral turpitude, is the most flagrant of them all.

In spite of having a personality of a tummeler, I practiced without incident until I stumbled upon the observation of mast cells in sinus tissue in OSA. My work in OSA probably started in 1990 and continued through 2005. Working under the radar, treatment was directed to patients with OSA. The light and electron microscopy at the University of Maryland, the surgical operations developed at Harbor Hospital, South Chester Medical Center and Philipsburg Hospitals, were carefully monitored. It was easier without an institutional review board. Also, my election as Medical Director for the staffs at Harbor and Philipsburg hospitals shielded me. I was transparent and open with the Board of Trustees, showing patients pre and post-operatively. And when jealous colleagues called into the Department of Health, my results were open for scrutiny. I was the only physician doing this type of OSA surgery and cured relatives of Board members. You will meet many of my patients.

Of course, BCBS of PA started with the printout and a new group of academic flunkies engaged to give testimony. It was 1977 all over again. There were no complaints. Of course, this was all under the auspices of the PA State Peer Review Society. Pending retirement and a beat up body didn't stop me from engaging the enemy. For some reason, unknown to me, all complaints were dropped. How strange?

This last surgeon operated under the radar. The innovator, the risk taker will always be scrutinized by jealous colleagues. Freedom works best. As far as respect from colleagues, rare. Rodney never got any.

CHAPTER 32

The Greatest Story I've Ever Told

Jonah was swallowed by the whale
This storyteller has finished his tale
There was a big boom
Two electrons collided at high noon
The Big-Bang released energy, gases and cosmic dust
Cooling of molten Earth created a hard crust
Matter was atoms of electrons, protons and neutrons
There was the first chicken quark soup with croutons
One and a half billion years ago
Viruses, bacteria, and fungi developed their logo
Gene sequences floated in the air
Ozone and antigenic particles filled the atmosphere
Evolution of innate and eventually adaptive immunity
Complex neuropeptides and cells presented a gated community
Immune cells were to fill the sinus void
Newberg unrooted the mast cell in the ethmoid
He traced sleep apnea to an autoimmune disease
Curing it was no breeze
The Medical Society nails innovative surgeons to the cross
They like to kill the albatross
This last surgeon fought a never ending battle each day
Truth! Justice! And the American way!

I was a teenage story teller. My cousins Lenny, Pam, Natalie and sister Nancy and brother Richard would listen to my tall tales before bedtime in Grandma's country house in Fleischmann's, New York. The stories were make-believe ditties. My spiel was to scare the bejesus out of them. I've come a long way to tell my never-ending story.

Sixteen billion years ago (bya) it was "bing-bang" after two electrons met head-on in a vacuum in deep, dark space. A gaggle of rocks, space dust, gases, and the energy from nuclear fusion including cosmic radiation would expand outwards. The universe was born. Billions of galaxies, solar systems and planets included Planet Earth. Finite matter of the Bang consisted of atoms. Quarks consisted of electrons, protons and neutrons. The word "quark" was confused with a ducks "quack." The quark made up "baryonic matter", mistakenly called "boney maroney" by me. The Boom had the sound of a low flying 747 passing over my house. The description of a space time continuum and gravities effects I leave to scientists like Albert Einstein, Bohr, Planck and Millikan.

The molten Earth was hot from nuclear fusion. So hot, that the helium and hydrogen were gaseous until cooling took place. Earths gravity was defined by Newton as an apple falling to the surface, or the pull of the sun on Earths orbiting the sun. It was so hot that the carbon in meteors and comets colliding with Earth became clear dense "rocks" that would be displayed in Tiffany's window. It was so hot that my mother could light up her ciggie on any of the planets orbiting the sun without a match. The expanding universe was a flatulent bubble. Breathing was difficult. Methane, ammonia and small amounts of CO_2 were present. The smells were comparable to the gases in the tailpipe exhaust of a running car. The cosmic rays would give a cosmic sunburn very nasty indeed. It took the ozone layer to dissipate the cosmic radiation to allow sunbathing in Miami Beach. It's been hinted that Grandma Essies chicken soup was a product of the Big Bang. We know there was a quark soup. It begs the question "was my mother there at the beginning?" The gene segments to build a kosher chicken evolved billions of years later with multi-cellular organisms.

The electron spinning in an orbit around the nucleus of protons and neutrons provide great distances between subatomic particles. The spin outlines the "dradle phenomenon", a subatomic dance trance. Is it this way or is it that way; is it up, or is it down? Did it move this way or that way. There is an electron cloud allowing electrons to roam in their nuclear orbiting playground. The amount of spin is always the same; in one of two directions. It has a definite axis of rotation in the process of measurement. Before the measurement you can't say where it is. You can't say it went from point A to point B. You can take a picture where it is, but you can't say how it got there. We know there is a certain potentiality—a tendency to exist. This probability pattern allowed atoms to exist as matter.

Physics at McGill University was a required course in the Bachelor of Science program. This freshmen course was considered a "killer." No one in his right mind would choose physics voluntarily. The quark with the subatomic particles of electrons, neutrons and protons was considered fair game. Just when you thought quarks were the end game, Quantum physics arrived. The quarks gave way to the gluons, mesons and pion; which were attracted to the quarks. The distortion of time – space (distance) and the effects of gravity was too much. I suspected that molecules were driven by a probability pattern. It's hard to imagine our atoms are determined by a crapshoot at the Borgata. Thank goodness for a grading curve; otherwise it was goodnight Irene, I'll see you in my dreams! I took Botany my second year. That's where a real man can express himself.

Cytokines are small glycoprotein's that modulate biochemical reactions. They have extreme redundancy and overlap other cytokines. They seem to have little specifity. The injection of five separate cytokines into patients led to organ failure. The cytokine storm in autoimmune disease like sleep apnea, mimics the excessive cytokines found in influenza. Young flu subjects die faster with multiple organ failures than older geezers. The "mature" patients have previous exposure and limited immunity from the H5N1 influenza.

When the mast cell belches it releases biochemical mediators histamine and heparin. Also, the enzymatic breakdown of arachidonic acid (AA) takes place. Ararachidonic acid, better known as mothers cod liver oil, was a disgusting foul tasting vitamin after breakfast. It tasted awful even when camouflaged in orange juice. This is a form of poison which would require a 911 call today. Cod liver oil is an essential fatty acid (EFA) affecting the health of a nerve cell. Besides a pathway to breakdown AA to express mucus from cells, the leukotrienes injure the ethmoid cells. The cytokines released from the AA are used to manufacture complex neuropeptides. These hormones are neurotransmitters that open ion and chemical channels in the neurons sheath. Schwann cells provide nourishment to the insulation (myelin) protecting the axon itself. Protein kinases are part of the neurons plasma membrane. They provide a bonding of the ligand or rubber band. They are reversible. The neural excitability and electrical messages are kin to a telephone line. These neurotransmitters affect the receptor sites in the neuron with other neuropeptides. A primer for the expansion of neuron receptor sites has started with substance P, and than neurotrophins. Neurotrophin growth factor (NGF) competes with neurotrophin-3 (NT-3) and neurotrophin 4/5 (NT-4/5). There is reversibility of OSA from the total ethmoid operation. Surgery reduces the mast cell population in the ethmoid. Raising the blood oxygen level in sleep leads to an improvement in excessive daytime sleepiness. Errigh LaBoo and the Seven Samurai, moderate to severe OSA patients using CPAP, underwent my sinus and throat surgery. The surgical cure rate for other physician OSA patients approach zero. Most University Centers will not operate on these severe cases. They refer them for CPAP. All eight patients presented in the book are long time cures.

The discovery of the fat gene, leptin in OSA is interesting. It developed from fat cells in the bone marrow, and resides in belly fat. It modulates fat stores in the body and plays a role in dyslipidemia and coronary artery disease. Raising the leptin blood levels should lead to decreased weight. What we see in OSA is a rise in the blood leptin levels. It appears that leptin competes at a competitive site in the brain. The receptor site is filled by neurotrophic growth hormone. This hormone causes OSA and causes misfiring of the neuron. We see this in sleep-disordered-breathing. The Restless Leg Syndrome is another neuropeptide competing at the receptor site. Again, misfiring of the nerve. Reversal of signs/symptoms of neurologic autoimmune disease is probable. The "Last Surgeon" chronicles the cure rate in OSA. Moderate to severe OSA cases chronicled here are 100% but on average about 85%. The cure rate for milder cases approach 100%. The reversibility of NGH must be compared with permanent nerve damage in multiple sclerosis (MS). This Last Surgeon is interviewing MS patients with the hope of finding clues. Knowledge and research are in too short supply today. My trilogy of the Anatomy of Autoimmune diseases including MS is on the front burner. The knowledge from probability patterns, relationships and interconnections of Multiple Sclerosis haven't been fully investigated.

Atmospheric antigens act like vectors for immune responses. The ability of our lymphocytes and mast cells to process antigens is not specified in the genome. The immune system is more than a genetic blueprint. There are proteins coded by genes, but it grows into something larger. By chance exposure to various antigens, the rearranged genes have responded to the environment. It appears that the children of OSA patients have atopic allergies. The addition of rearranged and modified genes may contribute to future OSA, obesity and high blood pressure. The new history of antigens and processing by lymphocytes and mast cells allows new signaling to enter the DNA of the marrow. Transcription and messenger RNA allows a different system of protein synthesis.

Immunity is built as a self organizing system. There is also the experience of interconnections and relationships. The immune system in space flight shows a weakening immunity. The weightless environment, vibrations from a weakening gravity on the genes, contributes to a weakened immune system. Diseases are more severe. The genes are not happy.

The cytokine nanonetwork (CNN) of tumor necrosis factor (TNF), interferon's, and interleukins form a unique and specific immune system. The system is built, and then it begins to learn. This becomes knowledge by experience. This knowledge may be harmful to our health. We are more than DNA because it's not capable of specifying all that we are.

Thank you patients for your help and support. You are those heroes. You are the greatest story ever told!

www.ingramcontent.com/pod-product-compliance
Ingram Content Group UK Ltd.
Pitfield, Milton Keynes, MK11 3LW, UK
UKHW060119300726
14090UKWH00002B/271
9781436365086